OSCEs and MCQs in
OBSTETRICS
AND GYNAECOLOGY

A SURVIVAL GUIDE

Commissioning Editor: Ellen Green
Project Editor: Sarah Keer-Keer & Jane Shanks
Project Controller: Nancy Arnott
Designer: Erik Bigland

OSCEs and MCQs in
OBSTETRICS AND GYNAECOLOGY

A SURVIVAL GUIDE

Joan Pitkin BSc FRCS MRCOG
Consultant Obstetrician and Gynaecologist
Northwick Park Hospital and St Mark's Hospital Trust
Harrow
Middlesex

Rory O'Connor BSc FRCSI MRCOG
Consultant Obstetrician and Gynaecologist
University College Hospital
Galway
Ireland

Chris Jenner BSc DGM MRCP(UK) MRCGP
General Practitioner
Elliott Hall Medical Centre
Hatch End
Pinner
Middlesex

Foreword by
R W Baldwin FRCOG

W. B. SAUNDERS
Edinburgh • London • New York • Oxford • Philadelphia • Sydney • Toronto 1999

W.B. SAUNDERS
An imprint of Elsevier Limited

First published 1999
  Reprinted 2000, 2002, 2004

ISBN 0 7020 2199 7

British Library Cataloguing in Publication Data
A catalogue record for this book is available from the British Library.

Library of Congress Cataloging in Publication Data
A catalog record for this book is available from the Library of Congress.

Medical knowledge is constantly changing. As new information becomes available, changes in
treatment, procedures, equipment and the use of drugs become necessary. The authors and the
publishers have, as far as it is possible, taken care to ensure that the information given in this text
is accurate and up to date. However, readers are strongly advised to confirm that information,
especially with regard to drug usage, complies with current legislation and standards of practice.

Printed in China
C/04

Contents

Foreword

This book will provide a survival guide for people studying obstetrics and gynaecology, particularly those doing the Diploma examination in Obstetrics and Gynaecology (DRCOG).

This book explains how to tackle and manage the DRCOG examination. In the past there has been a number of problems with the exam. These problems have led to changes in the MCQ section of the new exam, and to the practice of negative marking being discontinued. Problems with clinical and viva exams have been solved by the introduction of the objectively structured clinical examination (OSCE). This book will tell the reader what an OSCE is and what it entails: an assessment of professional competence and a test of knowledge and medical skills, as well as the ability to communicate. DRCOG exam questions are now standardized, making it possible to compare one candidate with another. The tighter marking scheme for the exam means that candidates are marked on 'an even playing field'. The transferring of exam marks using an optical scanner has led to a reduction in human variance, i.e. there is a reduction in possible human error.

Diploma candidates will find that this book offers insight into the setting of questions and the marking schemes used. When answering the questions it goes without saying that it is important to read the question thoroughly and to do what is asked, i.e. if four points are asked for, do not write a fifth. This book also gives the opportunity to practise in a timed situation, which is invaluable practice for the fraught position of an exam. Of course, students preparing for exams should not leave reading this book until the last moment, but should plan their revision and use the book over a long period of time leading up to the exmination, so that they are well practised in all parts. The good visual material contained in this book helps to make this a comprehensive revision guide.

Though this book will be of particular use to the diploma candidate, it will also be of use to undergraduates prior to their finals, and to overseas doctors coming over to take the PLAB (UK medical entrance exams). The book may also be useful to MRCOG candidates as this exam also uses the OSCE format instead of clinical exams and vivas. I am sure that it will also be useful to midwives as an aid to their everyday practice.

I hope that this book will help the reader to regard their exams as a chance to prove their knowledge, rather than as a hurdle to be overcome.

R W BALDWIN, FRCOG

Acknowledgement

The authors gratefully acknowledge a small educational grant from Wyeth Co. that allowed them to use colour photographs in this book.

WHAT IS AN OSCE?

THE OBJECTIVELY STRUCTURED CLINICAL EXAMINATION (OSCE)

Any assessment of professional competence ideally should test the knowledge, skills and attitudes required to fulfil effectively that discipline being assessed. The difficulty associated with any assessment tool is defining clearly what the examination is to test. Moreover, since examinations tend to dictate the curriculum, it is important to take great care whenever changing an assessment tool.

The place of the OSCE is now well established as a tool of both formative and summative assessment. Since its first introduction in the mid-1970s with undergraduates, its use has extended to postgraduate examinations. The Diploma of the Royal College of Obstetricians and Gynaecologists (DRCOG) was the first such examination to adopt its use, with other Royal Colleges intending to follow suit.

The OSCE is flexible and versatile. It has the ability to standardize a given scenario designed in such a way as to allow the assessment to focus on clear outcome objectives. For the newcomer to OSCEs, this is an important concept and candidates are always advised to put themselves in the examiner's position if they detect ambiguity or feel confused at any particular stage.

There are many 'tasks' which the OSCE can assess and readers will become conversant with these as they work through this text. Although this book is written with the syllabus of the DRCOG in mind, there is considerable overlap with undergraduate, midwifery and the MRCOG curricula.

When sitting an OSCE examination, candidates are encouraged to respond to the various situations as they would in the proposed clinical setting. In some instances this may be in the hospital setting and in others a range of community settings (Table 1).

Table 1 Possible scenarios for an OSCE station
GP consulting room
Telephone advice
A&E department
Home visit
Outpatients
Ward environment
Viewing data/results

There are a variety of tasks which are particularly favoured and targetted by those writing OSCE stations (Table 2).

Table 2	Clinical tasks conveniently assessed using OSCE stations
History taking	
Physical examination	
Communication skills	
Clinical interpretation	
Patient management	
Practical procedures	
Attitudes	

Communication skills are becoming a very popular focus for OSCE assessments in the format of interactive stations. The reader is strongly encouraged to revise these basic skills. Initially these constituted only 10% of the stations in the new DRCOG examination; they now comprise 30%.

The DRCOG

The new-style DRCOG was introduced in October 1994. It replaced the previous examination that consisted of essay papers, MCQs, vivas and clinical presentations. The intention was to create a new examination that would be more objective in its evaluation of candidates' abilities, easier and more practical to mark and would avoid potential examiner bias. There are legends suggesting that there have been examinations where two candidates of equal ability have had different examiners, one of whom is a 'dove' and guides the candidate through his initial nervousness and the other a 'hawk', who has had a bad lunch, is suffering from dyspepsia and takes out his wrath on the candidate. One candidate is successful and passes; the other fails. This cruel caricature has been a widely held belief, albeit an unfair one. Examiners have always aimed to be as fair and objective as possible. Nevertheless, there may be a grain of truth and like Caesar's wife, the Royal College has to be 'seen to be above suspicion'. Therefore, an objectively structured oral examination where all candidates are presented with exactly the same clinical information, the same specimens or the same role-playing interactive scenarios is now regarded as the best approach.

When restructuring the examination into the new format, the College aimed to incorporate more general practice-based topics. However, a certain basic knowledge of procedures occurring within the hospital setting has been maintained so that the practitioner has adequate insight and understanding of the subject to counsel patients appropriately. All questions are rigorously tested before they are used in the examination.

Introduction

The current examination

This is divided into two parts each lasting two hours: multiple choice questions which consist of 60 stems, each stem having five parts (i.e. 300 individual questions) and an objectively structured clinical examination. The OSCE circuits consist of 22 stations. Of these, two are rest stations and 20 are factual, problem-solving or interactive stations. Questions cover obstetrics, gynaecology, family planning, genitourinary medicine and neonatology.

The pass mark for each part is the mean score minus one standard deviation. Candidates must pass both parts in order to pass the examination. The MCQ paper is computer marked by optical readers at the College. The OSCE stations that are interactive or role playing are invigilated and marked by the examiners at each OSCE venue. The written questions are marked the following day by a team of examiners.

Initially there were only two interactive stations per circuit. Currently there are six. Some of these will be role-playing scenarios whilst others will be structured orals where the examiner adopts the role model and is looking for more factual information rather than a demonstration of communication skills. One examiner is assigned to each interactive station per circuit. Where possible, a seventh examiner will monitor candidates and the circuit as a whole. Examiners remain at their interactive stations for the entire duration of the session and they are given marking guideline sheets.

The stations are laid out in a clockwise or counter-clockwise direction, number 1 through to number 22. On arrival, candidates are given the circuit letter and station number at which they should start. They will be escorted to their individual starting station well before the commencement of the examination. As they sit down at their designated stations, they will notice an answer pack on the table in front of them. Each pack should have the candidate's name and number on it and should be opened at the appropriate page, i.e. the appropriate station at which that candidate is starting.

There are six minutes allocated to each station. At each station it is advisable to read all the relevant material before answering any of the questions or completing the tasks required. It is also important to restrict answers to the boxes provided and to put only one answer into one box. At the end of the six designated minutes, the bell will ring. The candidates must then stop what they are doing, leave the station, picking up the completed answer slip for that station and the answer pack for the rest of the stations and continue in the direction of the arrows to the next station. At the new station, the candidate places the completed answer sheet from the previous station in the tray provided, face up. It is then collected a few minutes later. At interactive stations, candidates are expected to wait at the holding point where they will be able to read the instructions for that station until called in by the examiner. Always check that the number in the top right-hand corner of each answer sheet corresponds to the station number at which you are currently seated. Because each station is different, it is imperative that the correct answer sheet is used for the correct station.

Practical points to remember

- Currently the examination is held in London and four other centres which are rotated around the country.
- All candidates are sent full written instructions before the examination.
- Candidates are expected to register by 10.15am at the very *latest*; candidates failing to register by this time will not be allowed to sit the examination.
- Evidence of identification must be provided, e.g. your hospital identity card, passport or other official document which carries a photograph.
- All MCQ questions should be attempted. Since negative marking is not applied, incorrect answers are not penalized.
- Half the candidates sit the MCQ paper whilst the others sit the OSCE circuit and the swap occurs at the end of the morning. At this time, strict invigilation occurs to prevent the two groups of candidates meeting.
- During the lunch break between the two examinations, candidates are 'held' in a waiting area. They are not allowed to leave this holding bay. Nor are they allowed to bring mobile telephones, text books, calculators or computers into the room.
- The afternoon session normally finishes by 4.30pm.

Most of the candidates questioned definitely preferred this style of examination to its predecessor and many found it quite enjoyable. In general, it was felt to be less intimidating.

How to use this book

Candidates are advised to read through the complete OSCE station before attempting any answers. By doing so they will get an overall feel for what information is required at the station.

Think carefully. If it appears that two questions require the same answer you can be assured that the same information will not be asked for twice within the same station. If one is asked to list the answers to a particular question, the examiners are only allowed to accept the *first* pieces of information given.

In this book the format of the Royal College examination has been emulated as much as possible. The layout of each question closely mimics the layout used by the Royal College. Whilst only three interactive stations are included in each circuit, it must be remembered that in the DRCOG examination there are six. Nevertheless, this will give the reader a feel of what to expect and also the opportunity to work through interactive scenarios with a colleague for some pre-examination experience. As many different types of OSCE station have been covered as possible – structured orals, interactive stations, demonstration of core knowledge, data interpretation and the ability to respond appropriately to given clinical situations. Generally, the current marking system of the College has been applied but in one or two places alternative marking systems have been used and these may be adopted by the College in the near future.

To get the best value from this book, it is recommended that you allot yourself two hours to work through an individual OSCE circuit. Having done so, you can check your answers and award yourself an overall mark. Comments have been provided for most questions. These have been based on the authors' experience in validating the individual stations. Furthermore, tips and pitfalls experienced by previous candidates are highlighted. It is felt that this approach makes the book more interactive and allows you to compare your efforts with your peers who have been involved with the validation process.

Many candidates are now sitting the DRCOG examination who have never done OSCEs in the past and others may face this format in their examinations soon. By working your way through the five circuits provided in this book you should have a good appreciation of this type of examination and, hopefully, will feel confident on the day.

These are exciting times and it is important that an examination reflects changing patterns of practice. It is even more important that the governing body is seen to be a vital, responsive organization and not merely a staid edifice. In view of the success with the new DRCOG examination, the College is now reviewing the structure of the MRCOG examination. A new style clinical examination, similar in structure to the OSCE, has been introduced to replace the current clinical examination and oral vivas.

The GP trainee

Obstetrics and gynaecology for those working in primary care

General practice has changed considerably in the last 20 years, catalysed by a number of important developments. The introduction of vocational training in the mid-1970s provided a workforce of general practitioners with better training and increased skills. The development of the purchaser/provider split and the evolution of fundholding has empowered some general practitioners to provide more clinical support in the community setting. Outreach clinics, improved surgery facilities and 'Changing Childbirth' have together made obstetrics and gynaecology a community discipline. The traditional secondary care placement of these units in some areas is no longer the norm. Clearly, for those requiring surgical intervention or complex antenatal/intrapartum care, this is still necessary. Nevertheless, for most women there is an expectation that their general practitioners should be providing an increased level of support. The Royal College of Obstetricians and Gynaecologists seeks to recognize this increased level of competence in awarding its Diploma, the DRCOG.

General practitioners are members of a wider primary health care team (PHCT) which may have all those working closely with GP surgeries as members. Midwives have established themselves as important 'partners' in this context. 'Changing Childbirth' has confirmed the important role of the midwife as a lead practitioner in antenatal care. The move towards a named lead practitioner and increased choice for the patient has also encouraged increased expectations of the PHCT. Those wishing to work in the community setting must be familiar with these developments including the role of the midwife, the expectations and rights of patients and the models of working in primary care.

This new delivery of health care demands that learners must be exposed to the primary care setting. New 'ambulatory' SHO training posts are being developed in some areas. These posts encourage trainees to cross the primary/secondary interface and understand in more detail the different approaches and skills required to deliver modern O&G care. Today's general practitioner is expected to initiate appropriate investigations and treatments in a variety of areas traditionally the remit of their secondary care specialist colleagues. Examples include the management of infertility, urinary incontinence, hormone replacement therapy and complex menstrual irregularities.

Finally, at a time when the curricula of many general practice-aligned specialties are expanding, there is also a need for GP registrars to gain more experience in the primary care setting. It is expected that in 1998 there will be a shift from two years being spent in hospital and one year in general practice to a new 18-month general practice attachment. As a result, the educational supervisors will need to ensure that adequate exposure will be provided to meet the above needs. Likewise, the trainees will need to ensure they take every opportunity to expose themselves to as broad a view of O&G clinical delivery as possible.

Getting the most out of your six-month hospital post

The entrance requirement for the diploma examination for obstetrics and gynaecology stipulates that you have to complete a six-month post in obstetrics and gynaecology. Most vocational training schemes (VTS) include six months of obstetrics and gynaecology in their two-year hospital programmes. There are certainly sufficient posts not dedicated to VTS schemes to accommodate those doctors making up their own scheme. It is probably important to remember when applying for posts that you are in a buyer's market. It is extremely difficult to obtain good calibre trainees to fill these vacancies. Your choice of post may often be dictated by geographic location but you should find out as much about the post as possible before applying. It is often a good ploy to discuss the post with the existing holder. If you are interested in securing a particular job, it is well worth discussing it with the consultant with whom you will be working, well before the post is advertised.

The composition of posts varies greatly. With a reduction in junior hours, many are now entirely based on a partial shift system though some on-call rotas still exist. It is important that any post that you apply for exposes you equally to obstetrics and gynaecology.

Within two weeks of starting the post, you should meet with your supervising consultant to define your educational objectives. The DRCOG working party reporting in 1992 suggested that all trainees should be assessed at two months, four months and six months. An assessment form outlines the knowledge and skills you should acquire during a six-month post. In most units, you will find your consultant supervisor will suggest meeting at three months and six months. Any glaring deficiencies identified at three months should be put right in the second three months. You may decide at the outset that some of the objectives suggested by the working party are not applicable to your particular situation. You will note that ten of the clinical skills are related to intrapartum care. Should you have made a decision not to provide intrapartum care in your future general practice, you may feel you do not need to be competent to perform such procedures as forceps delivery or artificial rupture of the membranes. Equally, you may consider that you require a greater proficiency in some gynaecological procedures.

There is always a dilemma in balancing service commitment and training needs. Senior house officers are required to perform procedures which may not initially appear strictly relevant to their future career. Procedures such as evacuation of retained products of conception are often seen as unnecessary for the average trainee. Nonetheless, they can provide a valuable opportunity to assess uterine size and instrument the uterus in a closely supervised situation. These skills will make practical procedures relevant to a career in general practice easier to perform, e.g. pipelle endometrial biopsies or intrauterine contraceptive device insertion. It is always worth remembering that enthusiastic trainees who are willing to provide the service commitment will probably endear themselves to their trainers and get more out of their posts.

Circuit A

QUESTIONS

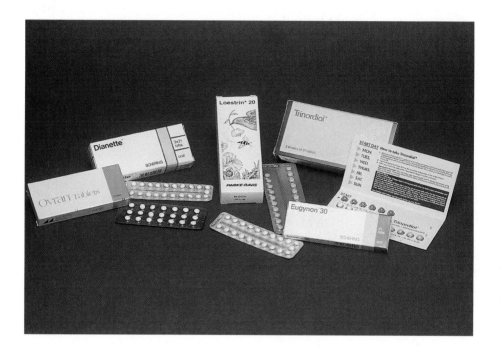

QUESTIONS

Study the packets of pills in front of you.

A► Which pill would you be most likely to prescribe to a 16-year-old with severely heavy periods?

B► Which pill would you choose to combat troublesome breakthrough bleeding (BTB) experienced with two previous routine brands?

C► Which pill would you choose for an epileptic patient?

D► Which pill would you choose if the patient complained of nausea, dizziness and cyclical weight gain when taking her current brand?

E► List three separate groups of non-contraceptive benefits of the combined oral contraceptive pill.

1.

2.

3.

F► Indicate three advantages that the new third-generation progestogens (desogestrel, gestodene and norgestimate) have over the old progestogens.

1.

2.

3.

ANSWERS/COMMENTS

Score

A➤ Loestrin 20

1

It is usual to use the lowest dose pill possible with a teenager and to change to a higher dose pill if there is breakthrough bleeding.

B➤ Trinordiol

1

Triphasics are best for breakthrough bleeding.

C➤ Ovran

1

Ovran (which many candidates have given for the answer to question B) is better for epileptics. A higher dose of oestrogen combats the fact that they are on long-term usage of hepatic enzyme inducers. Epileptics should also be advised to use the tricycle regimen (running three packets of pills together in a row followed by a shortened pill-free gap of approximately six days).

D➤ Eugynon 30

1

The patient in D exhibits relative oestrogen excess and should therefore be given a progestogen-predominant pill such as Eugynon 30 or Loestrin 30. Mercilon is the best oestrogen-deficient option.

E➤ Any three of the following:

3

1. Reduction in menstrual cycle disorders (including menorrhagia, dysmenorrhoea, premenstrual tension, ovulation pains)
2. Fewer functional ovarian cysts
3. Reduction in incidence of pelvic inflammatory disease
4. Reduction in incidence of ovarian and endometrial cancers
5. Reduction in benign breast disease
6. Reduction in trichomonal vaginal infections

Question E asked for three *separate* groups of non-contraceptive benefits. It is therefore not satisfactory to list dysmenorrhoea and lighter and regular periods as separate advantages since they all come under the one category of improvement in menstrual cycle disorders. We are looking here for examples from each of the different categories. Many offered 'reliability' as an answer, but the question asked for *non-contraceptive* benefits.

ANSWERS/COMMENTS

	Score

F➤ 1. More lipid friendly – minimal high-density lipoprotein – cholesterol ratio lowering — **1**

2. No effect on carbohydrate metabolism — **1**

3. Minimal androgenic activity (selectively progestogenic), therefore less likelihood of significant weight gain or acne — **1**

Following the recent pill scare that there was a slight increased risk of thrombosis with third-generation progestogens, this may be offset by their better lipid profile and lower incidence of side effects such as weight gain and acne. It should be noted that there is a sixfold increase of thrombosis associated with pregnancy.

 Howler! Smaller pill.

This question has been piloted several times, initally before the pill scare that occurred at the end of 1995. The original answer to question A at that time was Mercilon. The authors still prescribe this pill regularly to teenagers with menstrual problems, but currently the official teaching from family planning courses is not to prescribe third-generation progestogen pills as first-time pills. Therefore, to avoid controversy, the answer has been changed and the question re-piloted.

Many experts are unhappy that these excellent pills have been tarnished. Selection bias may well have accounted for some of the findings that suggest that the risk of thromboembolism is higher, especially with Mercilon. If clinicians are to prescribe a pill at all to an at-risk group then a low-dose oestrogen, third-generation pro-gestogen combination appears attractive. One source, however, does indicate that the slightly increased incidence of thromboembolism is genuine as the third-generation progestogens alter the oestrogen: progestogen ratio and create a relative oestrogen excess.

Currently it is safe to offer a third-generation progestogen pill if it is the patient's choice, if other brands of pill have been poorly tolerated (which may be the case in the adolescent age group) and if the lady is more at risk of arterial disease (family history or smoker).

The authors felt it appropriate to leave question F unaltered. There are definite advantages offered by third-generation progestogens for the abovementioned groups, which we should not forget.

QUESTIONS

E.D.D. BY SCAN **E.D.D. BY L.M.P.**

ANTE NATAL RECORD

Date	Weight	Blood Pressure	URINE Protein	URINE Glucose	URINE Acetone	Weeks of Amen	Uterine size in Weeks	Presentation and Position	Relation to Brim	Foetal Heart	Oedema	Haemoglobin Grms. %	COMMENTS and TREATMENT	Next Appointment in weeks
5/1/96	71	100/60	–	–	–	12	–							4
2/2/96	72	110/60	–	–	–	16	16	–				12.6		4
1/3/96	74	100/70	–	–	–	20	20	–					ULTRASOUND – NORMAL	4
29/3/96	75	110/70	–	–	–	24	24	–					HEARTBURN – GAVISCON	4
26/4/96	76	110/70	–	–	–	28	29	?		✓	–		GOOD MOVEMENTS ALL WELL	2
24/5/96	78	110/70	–	–	–	32	33	C	5/5	✓	–	10.9	GOOD MOVEMENTS ALL WELL SEE G.P. 2 WEEKS	
7/6/96	80	110/70	–	–	–	34	38.5	C	5/5	✓	–		AND HOSPITAL IN 9 IF NOT DELIVERED	

QUESTIONS

Score

Study the antenatal record card you have in front of you.

A➤ What problem have you detected?

B➤ List three possible causes for this.

1.

2.

3.

C➤ Name two tests you would have performed to confirm factors that might contribute to Problem A.

1.

2.

D➤ As her GP obstetrician, name two potential problems you would be worried about.

1.

2.

E➤ How would you manage this patient?

Perform a lecithin/sphingomyelin ratio

Yes/No

Arrange for induction of labour

Yes/No

ANSWERS/COMMENTS

Score

A➤ Large for dates. The patient has a fundal symphyseal height of 38.5 cm at 34 weeks.

1

The antenatal record card clearly shows that the patient is large for dates. Some amazingly interesting answers were produced by candidates!

 Howlers! *Wrong dates, mother thyrotoxic and overtreated, therefore hypothyroid baby; use of steroids; obesity secondary to overeating; a pelvic mass.*

B➤ 1. Polyhydramnios

1

2. Macrosomia

1

3. Undiagnosed multiple pregnancy

1

This question asked for the cause of 'large for dates'. A number of candidates gave diabetes. While it can be associated with macrosomia, not all babies of diabetic mothers are large. Others got lost in arguments about wrong dates but this is clearly not correct if you look at the antenatal record card. Similarly, some candidates argued about the answer of undiagnosed twins, commenting that the record stated a normal pregnancy on booking scan. However, twins *can* be missed.

C➤ 1. Ultrasound – will distinguish between all of the above

1

2. Fasting blood glucose *or* glycosylated haemoglobin *or* limited glucose tolerance test

1

Like question B, this illustrates the problem which can occur if the initial question is answered incorrectly, since subsequent correct answers are dependent on the initial one being answered correctly.

The tests you would need to request are those to exclude foetal abnormality or diabetes which are causes of 'large for dates'. Some candidates have suggested pelvimetry but this represents a quantum leap, making the assumption that the baby is macrosomic and then wondering if a large baby will deliver vaginally.

ANSWERS/COMMENTS

Score

D➤ Any two of the following: | 2

1. Preterm labour with potential respiratory distress syndrome
2. Preterm rupture of membranes with possible cord prolapse
3. Unstable lie (certainly true of two out of three and acceptable as an alternative)
4. Shoulder dystocia/cephalopelvic disproportion (true of macrosomia only)

We have been generous with this question by only asking for two potential problems. Whilst there are three possible causes of 'large for dates', there are several clinical scenarios that could occur and it should not be difficult to achieve two out of the four possibilities.

E➤ 1. No | 1
2. No | 1

In one examination, a surprising 25% of candidates wanted to perform a lecithin/sphingomyelin ratio and 50% wanted to organize induction. An L/S ratio might be of benefit in a proven gestational diabetic who needed early delivery. In this case, however, diabetes has not been proven and there is no clinical indication to induce.

QUESTIONS

Study the following indices of a 26-year-old primigravida who is currently at 30 weeks gestation.

	28 weeks	29 weeks	30 weeks
Serum urate	235 µmol/l	300 µmol/l	426 µmol/l
Creatinine	75 µmol/l	93 µmol/l	110 µmol/l
24 h urinary protein	0.8 g	1.2 g	3.0 g
Haemoglobin concentration	10.2 g/dl	10.5 g/dl	10.6 g/dl
Platelet count	212	180	120

A► What do you think is the problem here?

B► List three maternal clinical signs you would look for before deciding whether to continue to manage the pregnancy conservatively rather than proceed to delivery.

1.

2.

3.

C► You have decided that an ultrasound examination may give further valuable information. List three separate features for examination that you would ask for specifically on the request form.

1.

2.

3.

D► What three maternal complications can occur if the situation deteriorates?

1.

2.

3.

ANSWERS/COMMENTS

	Score

A➤ Pre-eclampsia, moderately severe   `1`

This is a data interpretation question and most candidates have been able to recognize the clinical problem.

B➤ Any three of the following: `3`

1. Systolic pressure more than 160
2. Diastolic pressure over 105
3. 'Small for dates'
4. Hyperreflexia
5. Clonus
6. Papilloedema
7. Liver tenderness

When asked to list three maternal clinical signs, it seems a little foolish to give an answer of reduced foetal movements and although abruption can be associated with pre-eclampsia, we did not think that vaginal bleeding was an acceptable answer in the light of the clinical picture created by the data given. This is quite severe pre-eclampsia at 30 weeks and as a doctor you need to decide whether or not to deliver, based on signs suggesting impending eclampsia and knowing that delivery will mean caesarean section. Induction of a primigravida at 30 weeks' gestation is not feasible and attempts would delay delivery. Some candidates thought it unfair that we stipulated the degree of systolic and diastolic rise, but in the context of a decision regarding delivery this is justified and your cut-off point needs to be specific.

C➤ Any three of the following: `3`

1. Diagnostic signs for oligohydramnios
2. An estimate of birth weight
3. Umbilical artery Doppler flow studies
4. A biophysical profile

Question C gives candidates the chance to show that they are aware of problems that can occur with the foetus. Many candidates have made the mistake of listing abdominal circumference, head circumference and biparietal diameter as three separate features whereas all three of those would be used to estimate the growth rate/birth weight and therefore detect growth retardation. The answer requests three separate issues for examination. Liquor volume and Doppler flow in the umbilical vessels reflect placental function.

ANSWERS/COMMENTS

Score
3

D➤ Any three of the following:

1. Eclampsia
2. Cardiac failure/pulmonary oedema
3. Cerebrovascular accidents
4. Disseminated intravascular coagulation
5. Renal failure/hepatorenal failure

The last question is straightforward and is used as an indication that the candidate is aware of what can happen if this situation goes out of control.

INTERACTIVE STATION

Instructions to candidate

You have a discharge summary in front of you regarding Mrs Jean Dolby who is 26 years old. She has made an appointment to see you in your surgery to discuss her recent management at the local hospital. She has one four-year-old child, Nigel, who has always been sickly. She has just suffered a miscarriage at eight weeks. Mrs Dolby will make several statements and will expect your advice and guidance.

GYNAECOLOGICAL DISCHARGE SUMMARY

Name	Jean Dolby
Date of birth	10/3/71
Hospital no	026743
Address	27 Carlton Place, Swindon
Consultant	Mr Bloggs
GP	Dr Tender
Date admitted	16/4/94
Date discharged	18/4/94
Diagnosis	Inevitable abortion
Operation	Evacuation of products of conception
Histology	Degenerating chorionic villi
Complications	None
Medication	None
Follow-up	To see GP in 6 weeks

....

SHO in OBSTETRICS AND GYNAECOLOGY

INTERACTIVE STATION

Instructions to actress

You are a 26-year-old mother with one child, Nigel, aged four, who has always been rather sickly. You have just suffered a miscarriage at eight weeks. You do not feel that you were treated at all well at the hospital and although you were in pain, contracting and bleeding heavily, you felt you had been left waiting in casualty for a long time. When you did finally see the young gynaecology SHO she seemed tired and preoccupied and gave many excuses about being busy on the labour ward and unable to come sooner. She also said that she had been on duty since 8.00 in the morning and had not even had any lunch.

When you were finally admitted to the gynaecology ward you were told that you would need to go to theatre for a D&C and you were kept nil by mouth for that purpose, but unfortunately you were never taken to theatre and nobody gave you permission to have anything to eat or drink. It was the next morning before you found yourself on a routine gynaecological theatre list.

You have come to see your general practitioner to outline these events and to ask his opinion as to whether you should lodge a complaint with the hospital management as your sister has recommended.

INTERACTIVE STATION

Score

Example of possible discussion

Mrs Dolby: Thank you for seeing me, doctor. I know you are busy, but I've known you for years; you've always been good to our Nigel and I can trust your advice.

Candidate:

Mrs Dolby: I am very angry and upset about how I was treated at the hospital. Have you heard from them? How much information have they given you?

Candidate:

Mrs Dolby: They don't care, you know – I was in pain, contracting and bleeding quite heavily, and I was waiting in the Casualty Department for hours. When I did get to see the gynae SHO, she seemed tired and preoccupied. Said she'd been busy with an emergency on labour ward – even though there were other doctors on duty, they'd needed her too. Then she said she'd been on duty since 8.00am and hadn't even stopped to lunch! Well, I didn't see her until 7.00pm. Why aren't there more doctors on duty? I don't want to see some junior doctor who's too tired and hungry to care!

Candidate:

Mrs Dolby: When they did get me admitted to the gynae ward I was told I would go to theatre for a scrape that night. Well, that was a joke! I was kept waiting all night, nothing to drink even. It was next morning when they finally got me added on a routine gynae list.

Candidate:

Mrs Dolby: It's not good enough! I've got little Nigel to think of. If I'd had my operation the same night I could have gone home next morning.

Candidate:

Mrs Dolby: Well, my sister says I should make a formal complaint to the hospital management. What do you think?

Candidate:

ANSWERS/COMMENTS

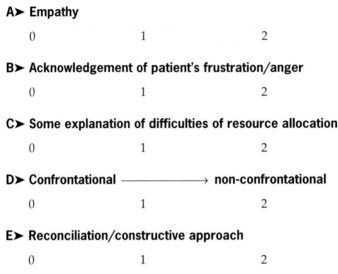

Score

Score is based on five modalities from 0 for poor, 1 for adequate, 2 for good.

A➤ Empathy

0   1   2

B➤ Acknowledgement of patient's frustration/anger

0   1   2

C➤ Some explanation of difficulties of resource allocation

0   1   2

D➤ Confrontational ⟶ non-confrontational

0   1   2

E➤ Reconciliation/constructive approach

0   1   2

This is an example of an interactive station testing communication skills with a particular patient type – in this case, the angry, indignant patient who wishes to make a complaint.

Primarily, you are scored on how you handle the situation, whether or not you can diffuse the frustration and anger and give some explanation of what may have happened, drawing to some reconciliatory conclusion in a reasonable period of time. Simultaneously, the examiner may well expect you to include some facts. In this particular scenario, facts are not so essential. You might comment that it is quite possible for junior staff to be delayed on the labour ward and if there is a major emergency, a registrar may require both the obstetric and gynaecological SHO at the same time. You might also feel it necessary to comment on her being deprived of food and drink that night and that at least she might have been given an intravenous infusion. Furthermore, you might add that you understand that sometimes acute surgical emergencies may have to go into theatre first and therefore these can displace less urgent cases like hers.

This is the type of argument that would be appropriate to present whilst trying to offer Mrs Dolby some explanation, simultaneously acknowledging her frustration. Sweeping aside her concerns heavyhandedly will not help the situation at all.

ANSWERS/COMMENTS

Score

The mock discussion we have included gives you an idea of how well these actresses may rise to the occasion. Bear in mind that they are university students and they are carefully vetted. There are usually more volunteers than actresses required. They also have a whole day before the examination to practise their role. You might find it helpful to work through a similar scenario with a colleague, taking it in turns to be either the actress or the general practitioner trying to diffuse the situation.

QUESTIONS

Score

A▶ 1. The caesarean section rate is trebled if continuous foetal monitoring with CTGs is used in conjunction with foetal blood sampling.

   True/False

2. 60% of abnormal CTG patterns occur in the absence of foetal hypoxia.

   True/False

3. A foetal pH of 7.22 at 6 cm indicates that the sample should be repeated 30–40 min later.

   True/False

4. Foetal pH is a good indication of chronic hypoxia.

   True/False

5. Blood lactate levels may also be used as an indication of foetal well-being.

   True/False

B▶ What is the normal range of foetal blood pH in early labour?

C▶ Name two precautions you would take to ensure that your foetal blood sample gave an accurate result.

1.

2.

D▶ Name two situations when it might be wise to use an intrauterine pressure catheter?

1.

2.

ANSWERS/COMMENTS

	Score

A▶ 1. False   1
2. False   1
3. True   1
4. False   1
5. True   1

In a recent examination over 75% of candidates answered parts 1, 3 and 4 correctly. However, only 9% were correct for part 2. In fact, 40% of abnormal CTGs occur in the absence of hypoxia. This is the reason why corroboration with foetal blood sampling is necessary. In the absence of foetal blood sampling, caesarean section rates would be trebled if CTGs were used alone. With foetal blood sampling, the caesarean section rate is less because we can identify situations where there is no hypoxia despite an abnormal trace. The answer to part 3 would have been ambiguous at a lower cervical dilation, e.g. 2–3 cm. With a pH this low and so far from full dilation, some obstetricians would proceed to section.

B▶ 7.25 and above   1

Several candidates got question B wrong because they had put too narrow a range, for example 7.25–7.30. This would suggest that anything above 7.30 was abnormal. Approximately 30% of candidates have got this question right.

C▶ 1. The sample must be obtained quickly   1
2. The sample must be pure   1

Question C has been answered reasonably well with 60% correct. Adequate lighting, precalibration of the machine and heparinized tubes are *prerequisites* of foetal blood sampling, but they are *not* precautions. It is particularly important to avoid contamination of the sample with liquor or meconium and to ensure that the column of blood is free of air bubbles.

27

ANSWERS/COMMENTS

D▶ You are allowed any two of the following:

1. Trial of scar
2. Breech presentation
3. Augmentation with syntocinon, in a multiparous patient
4. In an obese patient, where it is impossible to palpate contractions

Much to our surprise when validating this question, only 30% of candidates gave correct answers.

 Howlers! There were many: twins, abruptions, postpartum haemorrhage, uterine inversion and a cervix that was too narrow!

This question has now been piloted three times. At the last attempt, virtually none of the candidates had worked in a unit that used intrauterine pressure catheters. Nevertheless, the DRCOG examination must reflect general labour ward practice across the country. It is important to keep things in perspective: question D represents two marks out of a potential ten.

QUESTIONS

You are a partner in a three-doctor practice operating a 'personal list'. Mrs Jones, a lady whom you have cared for antenatally, has delivered a baby, Peter. The hospital has rung informing you of a six-hour discharge and as the paediatricians were not available to check the baby before discharge, they request you do so. Mother and baby seem to be quite happy when you arrive with your trainee to check them.

A➤ List two specific features you would be looking to exclude on neonatal examination of the following:

1. The hands

a

b

2. The face

a

b

3. The eyes

a

b

B➤ You are unable to palpate either testicle.

1. Would you refer?

   Yes/No

2. What advice would you give to the mother?

C➤ You are concerned that the hip creases are asymmetrical.

1. What might this signify?

2. How would you definitely exclude this condition?

ANSWERS/COMMENTS

	Score
A➤ 1. Any two of the following: absent or additional digits/horizontal crease; peripheral cyanosis.	**2**
2. Any two of the following: micrognathia; low-set ears; slanted palpebral fissures; cleft lip and palate; epicanthic folds; baggy cheeks; large fissured tongue; flat occiput; palpable 3rd fontanelle; jaundice. Haemangiomas and spider naevi (re Sturge–Weber syndrome) have been offered by one candidate out of three pilotings. We include this for completeness but logically it is best to offer *common* features associated with *common* problems.	**2**
3. Any two of the following: congenital cataracts (loss of red reflex); coloboma; conjunctivitis (gonococcal); congenital glaucoma; jaundice; Brushfield spots.	**2**

Unfortunately this is not a question that has been well answered. It is very important that candidates stop to read the question properly. In question A part 1, totally irrelevant answers have been given including undescended testes, congenital dislocation of the hips and bradycardia.

Several candidates have given facial palsy as an answer to question A part 2, which is extremely unlikely since you are informed in the stem that the mother had a six-hour discharge and presumably therefore a normal uncomplicated delivery.

 Howler! Fusion of lips.

Cataracts was not an acceptable answer here as there was a separate question on the eyes in question A, part 3.

Jaundice has been included as an acceptable answer for question A part 2 or 3. However, the examiners would be instructed not to accept it twice since there are so many other answers available.

 Tip: If your answer appears in subsequent questions or parts then go back and see if it was really needed the first time. It is unlikely that you will be asked for the same answer twice.

It was surprising that some candidates put epicanthic folds as an answer to part 3. Obviously, the epicanthic fold is skin and really belongs as an answer to part 2, i.e. the face. It is not acceptable for a question on eyes. Similarly, it is insufficient to offer 'red reflex'. It really is the absence or loss of the red reflex that is relevant.

ANSWERS/COMMENTS

	Score

B➤ 1. No   **1**
    2. Common finding; review at 6–8 months   **1**

 Differentiator: *Surprisingly, in one examination 28% of the candidates felt that they would refer if they were unable to palpate either testicle. This was an example of a good differentiator. Many candidates suggested a further check in six weeks' time, which is too soon, and others suggested waiting as long as a year.*

C➤ 1. Congenital dislocation of the hips   **1**
    2. Ultrasound examination of the hips   **1**

Ultrasound of the hip is preferable to an X-ray. It is possible both answers would be acceptable.

QUESTIONS

You are a GP and invited by the local branch of the National Childbirth Trust to give a brief outline of the 'Cumberlege Report' on maternity care.

A▶ What is this report otherwise known as?

_____

B▶ List six of the indicators of success cited in the Cumberlege Report that should be achieved within five years.

1. _____

2. _____

3. _____

4. _____

5. _____

6. _____

In the discussion that ensues, you are asked what alternatives there are to a home delivery for women who are not keen on full hospital care.

C▶ List two alternatives.

1. _____

2. _____

D▶ Is the perinatal mortality rate greater in the GP maternity unit than it is in a labour ward?

Yes/No _____

ANSWERS/COMMENTS

	Score

A➤ Changing Childbirth – How Maternity Services Should Be Delivered. — 1

Quite amazingly, in one examination 62% of candidates got question A wrong. One candidate put down 'Cumberlege Report' which was foolish since that was the title already provided in the stem. Others put down Natural Childbirth Report, Birthright and Maternal Mortality Report. Birthright was the charity fundraising arm of the RCOG backing medical research projects; it has now been renamed Well-being. Maternal Mortality Report deals with exactly what it suggests.

B➤ Any six from the following: — 6

1. All women should be entitled to carry their own notes.
2. Every woman should know one midwife who ensures continuity of her midwifery care – the named midwife.
3. At least 30% of women should have the midwife as the lead professional.
4. Every woman should know the lead professional who has a key role in the planning and provision of her care.
5. At least 75% of women should know the person who cares for them during their delivery.
6. Midwives should have direct access to some beds in all maternity units.
7. At least 30% of women delivered in a maternity unit should be admitted under the management of the midwife.
8. The total number of antenatal visits for women with uncomplicated pregnancies should have been reviewed in the light of the available evidence and the RCOG guidelines.
9. All front-line ambulances should have a paramedic able to support the midwife who needs to transfer a woman to hospital in an emergency.
10. All women should have access to information about the services available in their locality.

The emphasis of the Cumberlege Report is on reducing the number of visits to hospital clinics; it does not aim to reduce waiting time when you are in those clinics, although one would suspect if there are fewer attendances patients are seen more quickly. Again, reduction in mortality was mentioned frequently and is inappropriate. On average, candidates have been able to give only two or three correct objectives.

ANSWERS/COMMENTS

	Score

C➤ 1. Six-hour discharge   **1**

    2. GP unit delivery   **1**

D➤ No   **1**

GP units tend to deliver only low-risk mothers, hence the perinatal mortality rate is less than in hospital units.

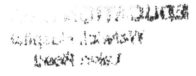

QUESTIONS

A▶ Fact file on fibroids

   1. Fibroids are present in 40% of women >35 years.

     True/False

   2. In Caucasian women they are associated with multiparity.

     True/False

   3. Hormone replacement therapy should not be prescribed to women with fibroids.

     True/False

   4. Fibroids can produce polycythaemia.

     True/False

B▶ List three situations in which fibroids directly produce pain.

   1.

   2.

   3.

C▶ Explain how fibroids may cause infertility.

D▶ Excluding menorrhagia, how else might a large 16-week fibroid present?

   1.

   2.

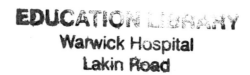

ANSWERS/COMMENTS

	Score

A▶ 1. False   **1**
    2. True   **1**
    3. False   **1**
    4. True   **1**

Question A has been answered reasonably well with just over 40% of candidates being correct on part 1, 60% for part 2, 76% for part 3 and 56% correct on part 4.

B▶ Any three from the following: **3**

    1. Colicky dysmenorrhoea, produced by pedunculated fibroid protruding through the cervical os
    2. Red degeneration in pregnancy
    3. Torsion of a pedunculated fibroid
    4. Malignant change
    5. Hyaline degeneration

One or two candidates wanted urinary retention included in the pool of answers to question B, as a cause of pain produced by fibroids. A posterior fibroid or a markedly retroverted fibroid uterus might give rise to retention by the same mechanism that a pregnant uterus can – incarceration in the pelvis. After consideration, the examiners decided against accepting this for B. This represents a more *indirect* way in which fibroids produce pain.

C▶ 1. Cornual intramural fibroid blocking tubal patency   **1**
    or
    2. Preventing implantation/placentation (accepted after review of answers)

Many candidates have offered recurrent miscarriage for the answer to question C. However, this is not an infertility problem. It is early pregnancy loss.

ANSWERS/COMMENTS

D➤ Any two of the following:

1. Pressure symptoms on adjacent organs, e.g. urinary frequency due to pressure on bladder, difficulty with defaecation due to rectal pressure
2. Abdominal swelling
3. Polycythaemia
4. Deep venous thrombosis

 Differentiator: *Question D tends to separate the good candidates who can think holistically from the average candidate. Most people would consider menorrhagia as a problem and this is why it has deliberately been excluded as a potential answer. Certainly, retention is an unacceptable answer for D as the stem has specified a 16-week sized fibroid uterus. By now the mass would have risen outside the pelvis and cannot, therefore, produce incarceration.*

REST STATION

STRUCTURED ORAL (Examiner is role player)

Score

Instruction to candidate

You are a family planning doctor doing an evening clinic in the local Family Planning Clinic. The door opens and a nervous young lady walks in.

Examiner's script

A➤ Girl: Oh Doctor, I hope you don't mind me coming. I've never been to see someone about this sort of thing before. Only my boyfriend and I are getting sort of . . . (sounds embarrassed) serious. I've been on the pill for three months now. I'm using up his sister's supply – cos she's stopped to have a baby. It is OK isn't it? (panic) I don't understand the pill, what do I need to know? I'm only 16 – you don't have to tell my mother do you? . . . She doesn't know.

Doctor (three aspects to cover)

B➤ Girl: I'm getting into such a mess with it – I never seem to remember to take it and with the three different colours if I forget one, I don't know which one to take next. (Looks hopefully at the doctor for guidance.) Can you give me any advice on how to take it?

Doctor (three suggestions/instructions expected)

C➤ Girl: If I miss a pill – is it all right to take it when I remember it? Is there a time limit?

Doctor (give full instructions here)

D➤ Girl: My girlfriend says that if I miss a pill near the end of the packet I might as well not bother and just have the week off then and there. Is that right?

Doctor (give full instructions here)

ANSWERS/COMMENTS

Score

Examiners mark for the content of answers regarding accuracy of information.

This station is an example of a structured oral. Here, the examiner pretends to be the patient and is expecting certain definite answers from you. The examiner will be given an outline script which will indicate that the patient is very young, very scared that her mother will find out what she is doing, has no idea what she is up to and has been borrowing someone else's prescription. The questions can be strung together in any way that the examiner wishes with as much padding as she wishes as long as the topics are covered. This station is designed to assess a candidate's ability to discuss the important facts of safe pill taking in an understandable and comprehensive way with someone who is quite immature.

The examiner, whilst checking that certain important facts are included in this discussion, will also take into account the attitude that the candidate adopts to the 'patient'.

A➤ 1. The patient is over 16 years of age. There is no need to tell anyone against her wishes. In fact, the code of confidentiality between doctor and patient is binding.   1

2. You would, of course, encourage her to be open with her mother and discuss her emotions and feelings honestly.   1

3. You must *not* sound critical and damning. She must be encouraged to see a doctor regularly and be properly supervised.   1

B➤ 1. Rule 1 – keep it simple! A triphasic pill is not a good idea for a young adolescent who is a poor pill taker; substitute a low-dose monophasic, e.g. Logynon 20, Mercilon.   1

2. Make a note of the day of the week on which she starts her first packet – she will always start a new packet on this day.   1

3. Link taking the pill to a set daily event, e.g. cleaning her teeth in the morning or bedtime drink at night. This will set a routine.   1

Question B has been poorly answered. Many candidates began to talk about injectables which, of course, were totally irrelevant since the question clearly asked for ways of instructing and exemplifying good pill usage. Others talked about what to do if the pill was missed, but that would only confuse the patient at this stage, since she had asked for advice on how to take the pill properly. She then proceeds to ask what to do if the pill is missed anyway.

ANSWERS/COMMENTS

<table>
<tr><td></td><td align="right">Score</td></tr>
</table>

C➤ 1. If only one pill is missed it may still be taken, if it is remembered within 12 hours. Take the pill and be sure to take the next one on time.

    2. If the pill is more than 12 hours late, the pill should be taken and the packet continued as normal but *extra* protection is needed for seven days.

Score: 1 *(item 1)*
Score: 1 *(item 2)*

Question C has been answered well, although there have been one or two candidates who felt that the pill could still be taken up to 24 hours after it was forgotten, instead of up to 12. Only one mark will be allocated to a correct definition of the time interval. Full marks will only be awarded if the seven-day rule is explained as well, particularly to a teenager.

D➤ No! If the pill is forgotten when there are less than seven pills left in the packet, she should start the next packet straight away, i.e. *not* have a seven-day pill-free gap.

Score: 2

Ten percent of candidates felt it did not matter if a pill was missed near the end of a packet. The lower dose pills certainly must not have a prolonged pill-free interval or rogue ovulation may occur. This is a complex but important point to include in counselling. It therefore takes two marks, an example of 'weighted' scoring.

This same scenario could be adjusted and simplified to be used as an interactive station with an actress playing the 16-year-old and the examiner scoring mainly for communication skills. The amount of knowledge required would be less than in a structured oral situation.

Tip: Some candidates complained bitterly during the piloting exercise that too many issues were expected to be covered in the time allowed. Remember, you are only meant to indicate to the examiner that you are aware of the topics and areas that need to be covered in this sort of consultation, not to give in-depth discussions on each section. The information must be accurate, however, or a teenage pregnancy might result.

QUESTIONS

Mrs Forbes-Smythe is a well-spoken 42-year-old lady. She is secretary of the local golf club and social secretary of the PTA, organizing their last dinner dance.

She is particularly distressed by urinary leakage that occurs mainly while walking her dog or during a round of golf. She is now reluctant to be 'caught out' on the links away from a toilet. It ruined the dinner dance for her. She is otherwise fit and well.

A➤ List five other urinary symptoms you would enquire about.

1.

2.

3.

4.

5.

B➤ List five specific categories of signs you would look for on urogynae-cological examination of this patient.

1.

2.

3.

4.

5.

ANSWERS/COMMENTS

Score

This is an example of a station testing clinical examination skills. Now that both the viva and clinical examination have been abolished, it is immensely important that an attempt is made to test clinical skills. It is surprising how badly candidates have responded to such straightforward questions.

A▶ Any five of the following: 5

1. Urgency
2. Urge incontinence
3. Urinary frequency
4. Nocturia
5. Adult enuresis/history of childhood enuresis
6. Hesitancy
7. Quality of stream (good, poor, interrupted)
8. Dysuria
9. Feelings of incomplete emptying, need to revoid

 Tip: It is so important to read the stem carefully. Many candidates have suggested they would enquire about neurological or bowel symptoms when they have been specifically asked to give urinary symptoms. Others have mentioned that they would enquire if Mrs Forbes-Smythe leaked with coughing but the stem already supplied the information that she leaked with walking and playing golf, i.e. on exercise, and therefore stress incontinence was implied. As 35% of incontinent patients have more than one problem simultaneously, this question was designed to examine the candidate's awareness of other urinary problems that might be present and their ability to exclude or confirm them on questioning. Some candidates suggested they would enquire about haematuria but this really gives no insight into leakage at all.

 Howlers! Vaginal discharge, recent weight gain and menorrhagia.

ANSWERS/COMMENTS

B➤ Any five of the following:

1. Signs of prolapse, cystocoele, rectocoele, cervical descent
2. Evidence of atrophic vaginitis
3. Can leakage be demonstrated?
4. Vaginal and rectal muscle squeeze power
5. Presence or absence of pelvic masses
6. Neurological assessment – especially including dermatomes S_2, S_3, S_4 and anal reflex

Unfortunately this question has not been answered very much better. Many candidates have offered cystocoele, rectocoele and cervical descent as three separate answers although they are all types of prolapse. The stem asked for 'specific categories of signs' – it is difficult to be less ambiguous. Some have proffered urinary tract infection as a clinical sign. Many have mentioned the pad test, but this is a method of measuring urinary loss rather than a clinical sign. Some people have discussed fistulae and others have mentioned chest infections. Obviously, coughing would exacerbate stress incontinence but is rather a secondary consideration and certainly not one of the primary clinical signs that one would look for on examining an incontinent patient. Also, the original stem indicates that this is a fit, healthy and active 42-year-old. A stem dealing with incontinence in an elderly patient who smoked would, of course, demand a respiratory examination. In one validation exercise, only 8% of candidates mentioned neurological examination.

QUESTIONS

Score

Charlene is a 23-year-old West Indian girl, whose blood parameters include:

Electrophoresis	Hb S/C
Percentage HbS	38%
Hb	10.5 g/dl

She suffered an ectopic pregnancy two years before. She is attending preconception counselling.

A➤ 1. She would like to know whether her risk of sickling in pregnancy is strong, moderate or weak.

2. Identify two risk factors that precipitate a sickle crisis.

   a _____

   b _____

B➤ What complications can occur in a sickle-affected pregnancy?

1. List two complications (excluding crisis) that can affect the mother.

   a _____

   b _____

2. List two complications that can affect the foetus.

   a _____

   b _____

C➤ This lady is booked for hospital care at 12 weeks. How would you manage this pregnancy? Outline three measures you would take.

1. _____

2. _____

3. _____

ANSWERS/COMMENTS

	Score

A➤ 1. Strong — **1**

2. Any two of the following: — **2**
   a Intercurrent infection
   b Dehydration
   c Hypoxia

B➤ 1. Any two of the following: — **2**
   a Recurrent UTIs
   b Renal complications
   c Haemolytic anaemia

2. Any two of the following: — **2**
   a Increased risk of miscarriage
   b Preterm labour
   c Intrauterine growth retardation

A large number of candidates have mentioned anaemia as one of the complications of a sickle-affected pregnancy, but quite a lot wrote down thromboembolic phenomena even though the stem had clearly excluded 'crisis'.

The majority included intrauterine growth retardation as one of the two complications affecting the foetus but a smaller proportion mentioned preterm labour. Many have suggested miscarriage as a maternal complication. While the examiners might have sympathy for this answer, it would not be accepted.

ANSWERS/COMMENTS

	Score

C➤ Either: 1

1. Maintain Hb A levels at approx 70%

or:

2. Prophylactic 'top-up' transfusions (3–4 units every six weeks). Some
   units operate exchange transfusions. 2

Then any two of the following:

3. Folate supplements
4. Serial ultrasound examinations
5. Serial midstream urine samples for culture
6. Maintain rehydration and prescribe oral bicarbonate (to increase
   urinary pH)
7. Offer prenatal diagnosis to exclude an affected baby/perform
   electrophoresis on Charlene's partner
8. Heparinization

The answer includes an example of a weighted score system. Management hinges on keeping oxygen levels high which necessitates reducing haemoglobin S levels to a minimum by the use of top-up or exchange transfusions which suppress marrow activity. Therefore it is obligatory to mention this in the answer to gain a mark. Any candidate who gives three measures from the list of alternatives but excludes to mention this topic will only be granted two marks. Folate supplements and serial scans were mentioned most frequently. Thirty percent of candidates suggested delivery in a specialist unit, although the question clearly stated that Charlene was booked for hospital care. It is more logical to test the partner first. If both partners are affected, the foetus is likely to be homozygous for sickle cell disease. Heparinization can be used in brittle cases to reduce the risk of bone pain, from both infarcts and thromboembolism.

QUESTIONS

Mary and John come to see you to discuss the results of their infertility investigations. All Mary's tests are within normal limits but John's semen analysis shows low motile sperm.

SEMEN ANALYSIS RESULTS

Volume	1 ml
Sperm count	10 million/ml
Sperm motility	20%
Abnormal forms of sperm	80%
Mar test	Negative

A➤ What percentage of infertility is due to a male factor?

B➤ What are the lower limit of normal values for:

1. Sperm count?

2. Percentage motility?

3. Percentage abnormal forms?

C➤ What two events in John's past history might give rise to his oligospermia?

1.

2.

D➤ What is the next step in John's investigations?

QUESTIONS

Score

E➤ What general advice would you give to a man with a low sperm count?

1. _____

2. _____

F➤ Would you recommend that the couple consider in vitro fertilization and embryo transfer next?

Yes/No _____

ANSWERS/COMMENTS

	Score

A➤ 20–30%

1

Even this question raised some controversy. A lot of candidates quoted the 'rule of thirds' – a third of cases due to male factors, a third due to female factors and a third mixed. Sperm defects account for approximately 25% of cases, whilst obstruction of sperm ducts accounts for 2% of cases.

B➤ 1. 20 million/ml

1

2. More than 50%

1

3. More than 50% normal forms

1

In validation this was poorly answered. A large number of candidates suggested sperm counts that were far too low; only 5% answered both parts 2 and 3 correctly. A semen analysis is a simple, cheap and very reliable test to perform, if done well. It is often performed badly and there can be tremendous variations in both count and morphology between different centres. It is always worth enquiring whether the laboratory you use undergoes external quality control. If not, choose a different centre. Computer-assisted semen analysis (CASA) has now been introduced in some areas. This enhances standardization, quality control and cost effectiveness by reducing technician time.

C➤ Any two of the following:

2

1. Mumps orchitis
2. Hernia repair
3. Excision of a varicocoele

> *Pitfall: Candidates listed drugs and alcohol. These are not events. They will only affect sperm counts if currently used and therefore are not part of John's past history. If John was taking salazopyrine and then stopped, his sperm count would improve in 3–6 months. We normally advise patients to stop smoking, reduce alcohol intake and stop all drugs that would impair spermatogenesis (e.g. cimetidine, salazopyrine). These measures often help.*

D➤ Repeat the sperm count

1

Before racing to spend money on expensive tests, the count should be repeated. Never label a man on a single sperm count. Intercurrent infections, stress and even jet lag can adversely affect a count.

ANSWERS/COMMENTS

Score

E➤ Any two of the following:

2

1. Avoid alcohol, drugs and smoking
2. Avoid hot baths
3. Avoid tight underwear

 Howlers! *Abstain from intercourse unless partner is ovulating; wash testicles in hot water.*

F➤ No

1

The question asked if the couple should consider intense assisted conception techniques *next*. It is possible they might be needed eventually but initially AIH (artificial insemination from husband) with superconcentrated sperm samples, AID (artificial insemination with donor sperm), IUI (intrauterine insemination) with washed centrifuged resuspended sperm should all be discussed first. Mary's tubal patency should also be assessed *before* planning the way forward.

QUESTIONS

A woman aged 46 years attends your clinic with a history of severe menorrhagia for 18 months. Her menses last 7–10 days with a cycle length of 24–28 days. She uses 'super plus' tampons, large sanitary towels and changes hourly on a bad day.

Frequently, she may need to take a day off work and has occasionally suffered 'accidents'. Her haemoglobin was found to be 8.9. Pelvic examination was unremarkable and ultrasound showed no abnormalities. Hormone profile was normal.

A➤ What is the likely diagnosis?

B➤ She is not keen to undergo a hysterectomy. How would you advise her?

1. Antifibrinolytics work well, with minimal side effects.

    Yes/No

2. Mefenamic acid could be used because it is a prostaglandin synthetase inhibitor.

    Yes/No

3. Noresthisterone 5 mg od from day 16 to 28 will work well in this case.

    Yes/No

4. Medroxyprogesterone acetate 10 mg bd from day 5 to 25 may be successful.

    Yes/No

5. At the very least, she should have a D&C and hysteroscopy.

    Yes/No

C➤ List three non-gynaecological causes of heavy periods.

1.

2.

3.

D➤ What surgical alternative to hysterectomy might be offered if all else fails?

ANSWERS/COMMENTS

Score

A➤ Dysfunctional uterine bleeding (DUB)   1

Usually this question has been answered reasonably well.

Some candidates offered hormonal causes to this lady's problem. The stem clearly states that pelvic and ultrasound examination were unremarkable (excluding anatomical causes) and that the hormonal profile was normal. This is dysfunctional bleeding by definition – an abnormal bleeding pattern with no obvious anatomical or hormonal cause.

B➤ 1. No   1
2. Yes   1
3. No   1
4. Yes   1
5. Yes   1

 Tip: Be specific.

Antifibrinolytics do work well – for a while – but often produce dyspepsia and diarrhoea. Therefore, the answer must be 'no'.

Similarly, noresthisterone can be very effective but in this low a dose, for only two weeks of the cycle, it is unlikely to make an impact on this severe a problem. (Noresthisterone 5 mg tds from day 5 to day 25 might help.)

 Tip: If a question (for example, Medroxyprogesterone acetate in stem B.4) asks if something may be successful or true, the answer is always 'yes'. Here, 'may' is a key word that should lead you in the right direction.

C➤ Any three of the following: 3

1. Hyperthyroidism/hypothyroidism
2. Severe anaemia
3. Coagulation defects, e.g. ITP, von Willebrand's
4. Anorexia
5. Stress/psychological upset
6. Obesity

ANSWERS/COMMENTS

Score

D➤ Endometrial resection or endometrial YAG laser ablation

1

Several candidates have suggested the coil as a cause of heavy bleeding in answer to question C but this could hardly be considered to be a non-gynaecological cause of bleeding and they have obviously missed the point of the question, which was to test whether or not a candidate could think laterally when a patient presents with heavy bleeding rather than just focus on gynaecological causes. Similarly, the progesterone-secreting coil was often given as an answer to question D. The Mirena coil does reduce flow but coil insertion is not a *surgical* alternative to hysterectomy.

INTERACTIVE STATION

Score

Instructions to actress

You are a 24-year-old single mother who has one daughter, Zoe, aged five with bilateral congenital cataracts. You had developed varicella at 18 weeks in your first pregnancy and had been reassured by the hospital that nothing needed to be done. Following this, you panicked in your second pregnancy and demanded a late abortion as you felt you could not cope with another child at that stage. Unfortunately, your third pregnancy ended in an ectopic.

You are currently 37 weeks into your fourth pregnancy and are demanding induction of labour, maybe because your nerves have snapped. The other added consideration is that your partner, Marco, spends a lot of time commuting between London and Milan and you are anxious to ensure that he will be present at the time of the birth.

You are pushy and demanding and want safeguards and guarantees. You are determined to have an induction.

Instructions to candidate

This agitated and highly strung patient is demanding induction of labour for no good medical reason in an otherwise healthy pregnancy at 37 weeks. It is the candidate's job to convince her that this is not necessary.

ANSWERS/COMMENTS

The examiner will want to assess if the candidate can take charge of the situation, that he/she can be sympathetic and empathic but at the same time remain firm and not seem to be vacillating from formed medical opinion.

Score is based on five modalities from 0 for poor, 1 for adequate, 2 for good.

A➤ Empathy

0   1   2

B➤ Acknowledgement of patient's frustration/anger

0   1   2

C➤ Ability to take charge of the situation

0   1   2

D➤ Professional stance – formed and firm opinion

0   1   2

E➤ Accuracy of medical information

0   1   2

In this interactive station the emphasis is on testing the candidate's ability to take charge of the situation in a pleasant, professional manner. It is extremely important that the 'patient' does not bulldoze the candidate and force him/her into agreeing to what is a social induction since the antenatal shared care card shows no obstetric or medical problem.

The candidate should include in the discussion the comment that induction of labour should only be performed if it is absolutely necessary and the medical team are prepared to continue to caesarean section if it fails. It would be kind to offer the patient a kick chart and regular antenatal outpatient cardiotacographs to try to ease her anxiety. The interview should end with a positive comment to the effect that her best chance of an uncomplicated labour and a normal delivery is if she allows spontaneous onset of labour.

Many candidates found this particular interactive station hard as they empathized with the patient's situation. The past obstetric history has been made particularly complex to see if this would sway the candidate's

ANSWERS/COMMENTS

judgement. In the final analysis, however harrowing the preceding events, they have no medical influence on the need/lack of need to induce. The patient is using them to some extent to gain sympathy for induction at a time when her partner is available. Some authorities would say this was a reasonable request, but the patient must be made fully aware of the sequelae of failed induction. Finally, the question has specifically stated that the candidate's job is to dissuade her. Sometimes the personal view of the doctor must be set aside and it is this ability to behave professionally and back the team/consultant's decision plausibly that is being put to the test.

You should try to work through this type of scenario with a colleague.

QUESTIONS

A➤ Outline two different situations when you might consider prescribing bromocryptine for lactation suppression.

1. _____

2. _____

B➤ Bromocryptine:

1. may cause retroperitoneal fibrosis.

    True/False _____

2. is contraindicated in cases of puerperal hypertension.

    True/False _____

3. interacts with Stemetil.

    True/False _____

4. should be started on day 3 postnatally.

    True/False _____

C➤ You are called to see a patient who has developed a fluctuating 8 cm abscess in the right upper quadrant. She wishes to continue to breast feed. Outline, in note form, three steps in the management of this patient and in the maintenance of breast feeding.

1. _____

2. _____

3. _____

D➤ What is the patho-aetiology of mastitis/abscess formation?

_____

_____

ANSWERS/COMMENTS

	Score

A➤ Any two from the following: 2

1. The mother has suffered a stillbirth or early neonatal death or late termination of pregnancy.
2. The mother is adamant she wishes to bottle feed but has a history of mastitis or breast abscess formation.
3. Breast feeding is contraindicated.
4. Child to be given up for adoption.
5. Mother is HIV infected.

Mainly answers to question A have included bereavement issues. However, candidates who have put down intrauterine death and stillbirth as two separate answers would only score one point as two *different* clinical situations are clearly asked for in the stem.

B➤ 1. True   1
2. True   1
3. False   1
4. False   1

Fifty percent of candidates have answered parts 1, 2 and 4 correctly. Only 30% gave the correct answer for part 3; the interaction is with Maxalon. Suppression must be started on day 1 as milk secretion has started by day 3.

C➤ 1. Incision and drainage (small subareolar elliptical incision, if possible). Leave a small drain in situ.   1
2. Mother to continue to express from affected side.   1
3. Baby to continue to suck from the other side. Re-establish breast feeding as soon as possible.   1

Some candidates wished to treat an 8 cm diameter abscess with antibiotics.

 Differentiator: *Obviously, the size was chosen deliberately. A smaller abscess might respond to prompt antibiotic therapy. This is large and fluctuant. Generally, however, this question was well answered.*

D➤ Entry of *Staphylococcus aureus* into the duct system, via cracked nipples. If there is stasis within a lobule, due to incomplete emptying, localized infection follows.   1

Most candidates gave the correct patho-aetiology.

QUESTIONS

Score

A 35-year-old housewife from Hong Kong, Mrs Chung, received clomiphene treatment for her primary infertility. A pregnancy resulted after six cycles of clomiphene, 100 mg daily from the second to the sixth day of her cycle.

The pregnancy progressed well apart from severe nausea and vomiting that occurred from the sixth week onwards. At 14 weeks, Mrs Chung was admitted as an emergency complaining of a reddish brown loss, present for 48 hours. On the day of admission she complained of heavier bleeding and cramps, yet still had pregnancy symptoms. Abdominal examination revealed a uterine fundal size equivalent to 18 weeks' gestation. The uterus was non-tender, but no foetal heart could be heard with the Sonicaid.

A▶ 1. What is the likely diagnosis here?

2. What other differential diagnosis would you consider?

B▶ If a speculum examination was performed, what might you expect to find in this case?

C▶ Indicate two tests you would perform to make a diagnosis.

1.

2.

D▶ Indicate three key steps in the immediate management of this patient.

1.

2.

3.

E▶ What advice would you give regarding future pregnancies?

1. What interval should elapse before conception?

2. What contraception should be avoided?

ANSWERS/COMMENTS

Score

A➤ 1. Hydatidiform mole | 1
2. Threatened miscarriage of twins | 1

A considerable number of candidates have had the correct differentials in the wrong order. Although it is tempting to put threatened miscarriage of twins as the most likely diagnosis, the patient is Chinese, a strong clue as there is a high incidence of molar pregnancy in China. She has had severe nausea and vomiting from a very early gestation and although she was admitted with heavier bleeding and more severe pain and there was no foetal heart heard on Sonicaid examination, she still had symptoms of pregnancy. Furthermore, it is unlikely the uterus would be non-tender if she was in the process of miscarrying twins.

 Howlers! Fibroids, ectopic pregnancy.

B➤ Blood and numerous grapelike vesicles protruding through the cervical canal | 1

Obviously, this question is an example of one in which the first part must be answered correctly in order that subsequent ones can be attempted correctly. Not surprisingly, candidates who thought twin pregnancy was the most likely answer for question A part 1 commented that speculum examination would reveal an open os or bleeding with clots. In one examination, 47% of candidates fell into this trap.

C➤ 1. Quantitative or semiquantitative, urinary human chorionic gonadatrophin (HCG) estimation (in a molar pregnancy an immunological pregnancy test is positive with dilutions up to 1 in 200)
or
Serum β-subunit HCG levels (also grossly elevated) | 1
2. Pelvic ultrasound | 1

ANSWERS/COMMENTS

Score

D► **Any three of the following:**

3

1. Induce miscarriage with Cervagem extra-amniotic prostaglandin.
2. Vacuum curettage to follow, to establish uterine cavity is empty.
3. Rescan at one week interval/re-evaluate as necessary.
4. Register patient on 'Mole' register to ensure careful follow-up at one of the three UK specialist centres.

Question C has usually been answered well. However, D has not. Many have commented that they would give the patient advice about contraception and future pregnancy, but this hardly constitutes primary management of a patient with this condition. These topics are covered in the answers required for question E.

 Tip: *As stated before, it is unlikely that you would be asked for the same answer twice. You should therefore always reconsider your answers if you find you are in this situation. Other candidates have put down counselling as an answer to question D and for similar reasons, this is not correct at this stage.*

 Howler! *Laparoscopy.*

E► 1. Avoid pregnancy for either six months or two years, depending on the patient risk status, as determined by the reference centre.

1

2. Combined oral contraceptive pill

1

Generally, question E has been answered well, although some candidates have suggested that the coil rather than the combined pill should be avoided as a form of contraception.

QUESTIONS

Score

Your patient conceived whilst taking medroxyprogesterone acetate 10 mg bd for 15 days each cycle, to control her dysfunctional uterine bleeding.

A► 1. What is the potential risk to the foetus here?

2. Outline two tests you could offer that might allay her fears.

a _____

b _____

3. Does the situation merit therapeutic termination of the pregnancy?

Yes/No _____

B► Malaria

1. Some parts of East India are endemic for chloroquine-resistant strains.

Yes/No _____

2. The risks of prescribing an anti-malarial are greater than the risk of malaria in pregnancy.

Yes/No _____

3. Folate supplements should be prescribed with dapsone.

Yes/No _____

C► Antibiotics

1. The risk to an infant due to the mother taking tetracycline whilst breast feeding, is as great as the risk of ingestion during the third trimester.

Yes/No _____

2. Maternal ingestion of sulphonamide increases the risk of kernicterus in premature infants.

Yes/No _____

3. The risk of deafness to the foetus is greater with tobramycin than with streptomycin.

Yes/No _____

63

ANSWERS/COMMENTS

These questions test quite difficult factual knowledge but these are the types of problems that come up in general practice settings.

A➤ 1. Virilization of a female foetus if given in the first trimester.   1
    2. a Detailed ultrasound   1
       b Amniocentesis   1
    3. No   1

Only 29% of candidates have answered question A.1 correctly. Despite this, they guessed correctly the tests that might offer reassurance – 75% mentioned ultrasound and 50% amniocentesis. Obviously, if the foetus is male there are no potential problems. Ultrasound cannot always be accurate, however, and amniocentesis may be needed, for chromosomal analysis.

Termination cannot be justified. Even in a female foetus the risk is small and any abnormality is usually amenable to surgical correction.

B➤ 1. No   1
    2. No   1
    3. Yes   1

    1. 40% answered correctly.

 Differentiator: The answer was West India.

    2. 80% answered correctly. (The risk of malarial-induced miscarriage is greater.)
    3. 80% answered correctly.

C➤ 1. No   1
    2. Yes   1
    3. No   1

    1. 60% answered correctly. (Theoretically, milk proteins chelate the tetracycline.)
    2. 76% answered correctly.
    3. 84% answered correctly.

QUESTIONS

Score

A➤ 1. What is the cause of toxic shock syndrome (TSS)?

2. What is the most common gynaecological cause?

3. What is the mortality rate?

%

B➤ List three possible complications of acute TSS.

1.

2.

3.

C➤ Some cases of TSS are related to menstruating women using tampons.

1. How would you recognize the illness? Indicate how it presents clinically.

2. If a female patient is worried, give three pieces of advice regarding the safe use of tampons.

a

b

c

ANSWERS/COMMENTS

	Score

A➤ 1. A staph aurens exotoxin (also known as toxic shock syndrome toxin-1)   **1**
2. Septic abortion
3. Still in the order of 5–15%

    1
    1

The majority of candidates seemed to feel that either streptococcus or staphylococcus was the cause of toxic shock syndrome. It was also felt that 'lost tampons' was a commoner cause of toxic shock than septic abortion. Forty-six percent of candidates were correct in the order of mortality that occurs with this clinical condition.

B➤ Any three of the following:

   1. Venous poisoning with reduced cardiac return, fall in cardiac output   **3**
      and BP
   2. Tissue, hypoxia
   3. Increased capillary permeability
   4. Disseminated intravascular coagulation (DIC)
   5. Renal tubal or cortical necrosis
   6. Microthrombi
   7. Adult respiratory distress syndrome (ARDS)

Since we had only asked for three possible complications of acute TSS and there were seven to choose from, we felt this was a fairly generous option. We did not think that infertility was an acceptable answer, since we had asked for complications of the acute situation and we felt that candidates who offered death as an answer were being a little facetious.

ANSWERS/COMMENTS

Score

C➤ 1. Flu-like symptoms with high fever – 39°C (102°F) – diarrhoea, vomiting, rash, muscle aches, offensive discharge

1

2. Any three of the following:
   - a Use the lowest absorbency tampon suitable for the individual's flow.
   - b Change tampons every 4–8 hours.
   - c Wash hands before and after insertion.
   - d Remove tampon at end of menses.

3

Question C was designed to test the candidate's ability to recognize this uncommon but serious condition and to be able to give useful common-sense advice on how to avoid this, which is something that a family doctor may be called upon to do.

Howlers!
If it goes in it must come out!
Don't use overnight!
Must remove before inserting the next one!
Use tampons that fit!

We must add that these howlers came from candidates of both sexes and were not predominantly confined to the male GP trainees.

REST STATION

QUESTIONS

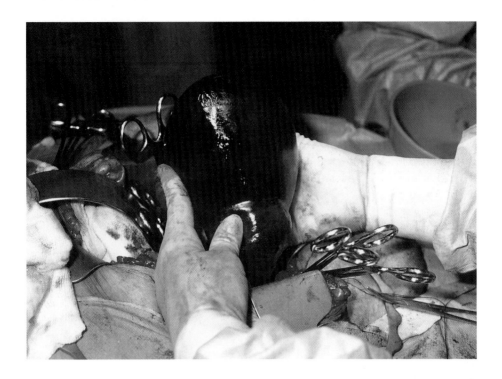

QUESTIONS

A► Study the photograph in front of you.

   1. What does it show?

   2. What complication might follow?

B► List two investigations you would perform after clinically eliciting a pelvic mass in a 50-year-old.

   1.

   2.

C► In any 50-year-old, list three possible different diagnoses of a pelvic mass.

   1.

   2.

   3.

D► 1. There is a significant increased risk of ovarian epithelial cancer in women reporting thyroid carcinoma in first-degree relatives.

   True/False

   2. The death rate from ovarian carcinoma in the UK is now 13 000 per annum.

   True/False

   3. There is an association between social class and incidence of ovarian cancer.

   True/False

ANSWERS/COMMENTS

	Score

A➤ 1. Torted ovarian cyst. This proved to be a benign cyst, torted six times on its pedicle.   **1**

2. Rupture. This can produce shock and peritonitis. The contents of chocolate and dermoid cysts are extremely irritant and may cause severe symptoms.   **1**

1. While 50% of candidates have identified the structure as an ovarian cyst, only half of these said it was torted. This information is required to gain the mark. The photograph shows a purple-black mass, so the diagnosis is obvious.
2. Sadly, 25% of candidates have opted for torsion. If one looks at the photograph, one will see that this has already occurred. The question asks what complication might *follow*.

Many candidates showed no comprehension and listed general postoperative complications.

B➤ Any two of the following: **2**

1. Pelvic ultrasound or pelvic CAT scan
2. Intravenous pyelogram or renal ultrasound
3. CA 125
4. Barium enema

Only a third of candidates have managed to give the correct investigation despite the long list of acceptable ones. Many have wanted to perform a laparoscopy which would be potentially dangerous, risking puncture and dissemination of a malignancy. Fifteen percent have wanted to undertake a hysteroscopy or endometrial biopsy. This would provide no useful information. The score system has been adjusted to prevent offering two tests that perform the same function, e.g. IVU and renal scan.

ANSWERS/COMMENTS

Score
3

C➤ Any three of the following:

1. Fibroids
2. Ovarian neoplasm, either benign or malignant
3. Full bladder
4. Pelvic or polycystic kidney
5. Tumour of colon or rectum
6. Retroperitoneal tumour
7. Hydronephrosis

The majority of candidates have offered two correct suggestions. Endometrial carcinoma and cervical carcinoma, suggested by many, are very unlikely to give rise to a pelvic mass and are therefore not acceptable. Several candidates have given different varieties of ovarian carcinoma which will not be accepted. The question asked for 'three possible *different* diagnoses'. Although IVF-assisted pregnancies have been reported in menopausal women, using donor eggs, pregnancy is not an acceptable answer here. The question is obviously looking at differential diagnoses of a pelvic mass (e.g. possible malignancy) and there are seven suitable alternatives to choose from.

D➤ 1. False   1
    2. False   1
    3. True   1

 Differentiator: *Only 15% of candidates have all three correct. Part 1 had the least number of correct answers and part 3 the most.*

1. The association is between epithelial ovarian carcinoma and first-degree relatives with breast or colorectal cancer.
2. The death rate currently stands at approximately 3800 per annum. Breast cancer accounts for approximately 13 000 deaths per annum.
3. Mortality from ovarian cancer in class I is twice that in class V.

QUESTIONS

A 30-year-old woman with poorly controlled epilepsy treated with phenobarbitone and phenytoin is planning her first pregnancy. She understands from advice given previously that it is important she discuss this with you.

A➤ She has a number of concerns and asks the following questions.

    1. What can she do to help control her epilepsy during pregnancy?

      a

      b

    2. What specific measures will you, as the doctor, take to optimize control in pregnancy?

      a

      b

B➤ 1. What specific abnormality is the foetus at risk of if she continues with her *current* medication?

    2. What might be a more appropriate antiepileptic to use in pregnancy?

C➤ If you change to this *alternative* anticonvulsant:

    1. What *specific* foetal anomaly may occur then?

    2. What test could you offer for reassurance?

    3. What measure may prevent this problem arising?

D➤ Is the untreated epileptic at increased risk of foetal abnormalities?

    Yes/No

ANSWERS/COMMENTS

	Score

A▶ 1. a Good compliance — **1**
  b Avoid stress/flashing lights — **1**
 2. Any two of the following: — **2**
  a Monitor drug levels
  b Change to more appropriate therapy
  c Refer to combined obstetrician-physician high-risk antenatal clinic

1. Just over 50% of the candidates mentioned compliance, i.e. regularly taking her medication during pregnancy.

 Pitfall: *Several fell into the trap of stressing the need for good control **prior** to conception. Although this is a valid point, the question clearly asked for what she could do to help control **during** pregnancy.*

Only approximately one third of candidates mentioned the need to avoid stress.

2. Over 90% recognized the need to monitor blood levels.

Amazingly, *no-one* suggested changing the medication and only two candidates referred to the concept of conjoint (combined obstetrician-physician) clinics.

 Howler! *Prompt treatment for raised blood pressure, though necessary in its own right, was not **specific** to this problem.*

B▶ 1. Cleft lip and palate — **1**
 2. Carbamazepine or sodium valproate — **1**

1. Surprisingly, there were several offerings of congenital heart disease. Just over half the candidates mentioned foetal hydantoin syndrome (i.e. cleft lip and palate).
2. Everyone was correct; the majority preferred carbamazepine.

ANSWERS/COMMENTS

	Score
C➤ 1. Spinal abnormality	1
2. Ultrasound or amniocentesis for acetylcholinesterase levels	1
3. Folic acid three months before conception and first three months of pregnancy	1

1. There was obviously considerable confusion over this point, many candidates considering cleft lip to be the specific defect. Just over half were correct.
2. Ultrasound is the specific test here. Serum α-fetoprotein can be raised for other reasons. The two may be used in conjunction.

   Amniotic fluid acetylcholinesterase levels are specific but require an invasive procedure (amniocentesis), carrying a 1% miscarriage rate. The answer, however, is not incorrect.

D➤ Yes

The majority of candidates have answered both the last two questions (C and D) correctly.

1

Circuit B

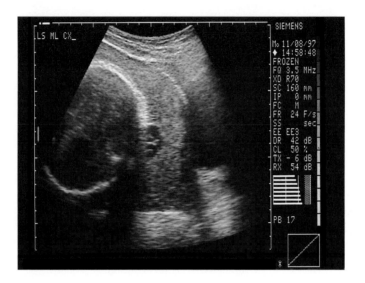

QUESTIONS

Study the scan in front of you of a 31-week gestation primip.

A➤ 1. Report the salient ultrasound features.

2. What is your diagnosis?

The patient presents to the labour ward without the scan after a painless bleed of approximately two cupfuls of blood whilst in a supermarket.

B➤ Concerning your management, would you:

1. perform an internal examination?

   Yes/No

2. perform a speculum examination?

   Yes/No

3. rescan the patient in ten days?

   Yes/No

4. keep this patient in until delivery?

   Yes/No

C➤ After what stage is the lower uterine segment fully formed?

D➤ List the two clinical features most likely to influence your future management of delivery (excluding foetal distress) at term.

1.

2.

E➤ What is the worrying feature of a vasa praevia?

ANSWERS/COMMENTS

	Score

A➤ 1. The patient's scan shows the tongue of placental tissue beside the foetal head but 4–5 cm from the internal os.   **1**

2. Placenta praevia grade 1   **1**

Many candidates have given placenta praevia but only 30% added that the photograph showed a grade 1 praevia. The key point to notice is that the placenta is not in front of the baby's head, i.e. not covering the os.

 Howlers! *Normal-sized foetus, 31-week foetus – hardly! It is in the stem.*

B➤ 1. No   **1**
    2. Yes   **1**
    3. No   **1**
    4. No   **1**

Most clinicians perform speculum examinations as other vaginal causes of bleeding can be present, e.g. a polyp, and cervical dilation must be assessed. This is not controversial but caused alarm with some candidates during validation. Ten days is too soon to perform another scan as the placenta will not have migrated in such a short time. It is reasonable to allow a woman with a grade 1 praevia home after 3–4 days if she has no further bleeding. If it had been a grade 4 praevia, admission until delivery would be the norm.

C➤ 34 weeks   **1**

Candidates have given quite a range here.

 Howlers! *18 weeks, second stage of labour.*

D➤ 1. Further episodes of bleeding (especially if heavy)   **1**
    2. If the head remains unengaged at term   **1**

The majority of candidates have suggested bleeding; only a few mentioned a high head at term. The issue is, of course, continued repeated bleeds or a heavy bleed, defined as over 500 ml. Most primigravidae engage between 34 and 37 weeks' gestation. If the head remains unengaged at term then suspicions must be raised that the degree of praevia is greater than originally reported.

ANSWERS/COMMENTS

Score

1

E➤ Foetal blood rather than maternal blood is being lost although it presents as painless bleeding.

In a vasa praevia, a large vessel lies on the membranes just above the cervix. If these tear, a large foetal bleed can occur.

 Howlers! Placenta invades into the uterine myometrium (this is a placenta accreta); maternal death (only fetal blood is lost).

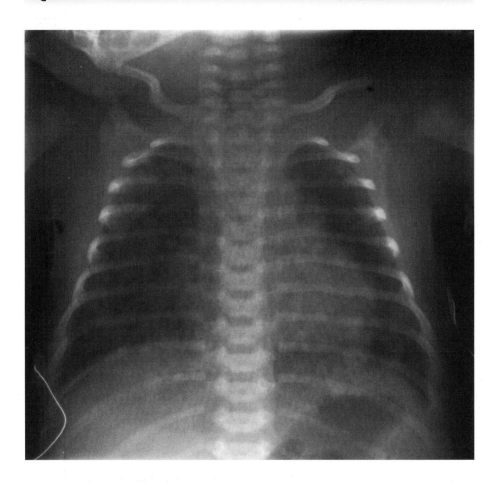

QUESTIONS

Score

A➤ 1. What do you understand by the term grade 1 meconium?

2. What is the significance of its presence?

3. What do you understand by the term grade 3 meconium?

B➤ 1. Meconium is present in 30% of all term deliveries.

True/False

2. Absence of meconium in labour at 30 weeks' gestation does not exclude hypoxia.

True/False

3. During labour at 41 + 5 weeks' gestation, fresh meconium, even with a normal cardiotocography trace, is an indication for foetal blood sampling.

True/False

C➤ Study the X-ray in front of you. What does it show?

D➤ List three practical ways in which you could take steps to prevent the situation in this X-ray occurring at the time of delivery.

1.

2.

3.

ANSWERS/COMMENTS

	Score

A➤ 1. Old meconium – liquor usually a pale yellow-brown colour   **1**
2. May indicate previous (i.e. prepartum) in utero distress   **1**
3. Fresh meconium – thick, pea-green and opaque   **1**

This may be regarded by some as controversial. Not all obstetric units grade meconium. Old meconium is important because it may be associated with long-standing hypoxia which may lead to developmental delay in childhood. Candidates have confused grades 1 and 3.

B➤ 1. False   **1**
2. True   **1**
3. False   **1**

Well answered apart from part 1. Meconium is present in 5–10% of *all* deliveries. A 30-week foetus is too immature to produce meconium as a response to stress. Thirty percent of postmature babies produce meconium but its presence does not always signify distress. Foetal blood sampling should only be performed if the cardiotocograph tracing is abnormal.

C➤ Meconium aspiration syndrome (blotchy shadowing and   **1**
hyperinflated lungs)

In one examination, 45% of candidates answered respiratory distress syndrome. This is an unlikely answer considering that the station focuses on meconium.

D➤ Three of the following are allowed: **3**

1. Suck out the nasopharynx as soon as the baby's head is delivered.
2. As soon as the delivery has occurred, check that no aspiration below the cords has occurred, i.e. by direct vision laryngoscopy.
3. If meconium is present, intubate and apply suction.
4. Whenever there is meconium staining of the amniotic fluid, ensure someone skilled in intubation is present at delivery.

If question C was not answered correctly the candidate missed out on this question also. In one sitting of this question there was controversy as to whether the nasopharynx should be sucked out as the head is delivered. It was argued that this would stimulate the baby to gasp and any meconium on the cords would be inhaled. However, the baby usually cries on reaching air. Suction prevents more meconium being aspirated that might otherwise be the case.

QUESTIONS

You are one of five GP obstetricians who cover a local low-risk GP delivery unit. You are 'crash-bleeped' to attend by a very experienced community midwife who has been supervising Mrs Brannigan's delivery. Mrs Brannigan has had three previous normal deliveries; birth weights 7 lb 5 oz, 7 lb 13 oz and 8 lb 13oz. This pregnancy was uneventful and she had mainly GP antenatal care with only two hospital visits (booking and 34 weeks). She went into spontaneous labour at 41 weeks and progressed well. When you last phoned she was 8 cm dilated. On arrival, you noted Mrs Brannigan, lying on a delivery bed, knees flexed and bearing down. The head had delivered but was a dusky blue. The midwife was applying suprapubic pressure. The perineum is intact.

A➤ State your immediate actions in this case.

1.

2.

3.

B➤ Your initial efforts have failed. State in the correct sequence the next three manoeuvres you would try.

1.

2.

3.

C➤ Reviewing Mrs Brannigan's case, list two antenatal tests that should have been performed.

1.

2.

D➤ State two ways in which the management of this delivery could have been improved if the problems had been anticipated.

1.

2.

ANSWERS/COMMENTS

	Score

A➤ 1. Maximally flex legs/place patient in lithotomy. **1**
2. Cut episiotomy. **1**
3. Apply truncal flexion, whilst midwife continues suprapubic pressure. **1**

It is essential that you are familiar with the management of shoulder dystocia in an obstetric emergency. We suggest you review the answer provided again and read an account of the management in a standard text book. Many candidates said as an SHO they would call the registrar but in this scenario you are a GP in a GP unit and you have no-one to call. There would not be time to call the flying squad, as some candidates have suggested.

 Howlers! *Introducing yourself; give oxygen to the mother; over 70% of candidates said check if the cord was around the neck – the midwife would have done this before she attempted to deliver the shoulders!*

B➤ 1. Cut second episiotomy. **1**
2. Fracture fetal clavicles. **1**
3. Perform symphysiotomy. **1**

 Howlers! *Lift out forceps; cut cord.*

Only 10% of candidates have suggested fracture of the clavicle and 5% symphysiotomy.

C➤ 1. Glucose tolerance test/random glucose **1**
2. Ultrasound for estimated weight **1**

Reviewing the history given, Mrs Brannigan's three previous babies all had steadily increasing birth weights. Gestational diabetes may have been missed here and no-one has suspected the size of this infant.

D➤ Any two of the following: **2**

1. If a big baby is suspected, deliver in the maternity unit of the local hospital.
2. Have a doctor present for delivery.
3. Prophylactic episiotomy

You must include no. 3 and either 1 or 2.

QUESTIONS

Score

Mrs Peters is 39 years of age and has made an appointment to see you following a recent outpatient appointment at the gynaecology clinic. She has been recommended to have a hysterectomy for menorrhagia. The previous D&Cs have shown no sinister pathology and she is known to have a 16-week fibroid uterus. Mrs Peters is requesting a second opinion as her neighbour (who has had 'similar problems') tells her that she should have the new 'laser treatment'.

A➤ 1. What was the 'laser treatment' her neighbour had?

2. Name two other non-laparoscopic, minimally invasive surgical procedures you know for menorrhagia.

a

b

B➤ Would Mrs Peters be suitable for this 'laser treatment'?

Yes/No

C➤ In counselling a patient about 'laser treatment':

1. What percentage of patients continue to bleed?

%

2. Do they need subsequent contraception?

Yes/No

3. When these patients become menopausal, do they require progestogens as well as oestrogens for HRT?

Yes/No

QUESTIONS

D► Which of the alternatives would be suitable methods of treatment for Mrs Peters' problems?

1. Progestogen therapy

   Yes/No

2. Vaginal hysterectomy

   Yes/No

3. Laparoscopic-assisted vaginal hysterectomy

   Yes/No

ANSWERS/COMMENTS

	Score

A➤ 1. YAG endometrial laser ablation   **1**

     2. Any two of the following: **2**

        a   Endometrial resection

        b   Rollerball

        c   Radiofrequency endometrial ablation

        d   Thermal ablation

     1. Many candidates have given transcervical resection of the endometrium but this is performed using a hot resectional loop, not a laser.

     !?! *Howlers! Treatment for cervical carcinoma, myomectomy.*

     2. The question asked for surgical procedures. Insertion of a progestogen-secreting IUCD would not be accepted. Dilatation and curettage was offered by many, but this is a diagnostic procedure and not a therapeutic one.

B➤ No   **1**

C➤ 1. 15–30%   **1**

     2. Yes   **1**

     3. Yes   **1**

Mrs Peters will need contraception following the procedure. She is only 39 years of age and her endometrium may regenerate. Laparoscopic sterilization may be performed at the same time. Some centres are now inserting tubal plugs.

Pockets of endometrium can be left in the uterus or can regenerate, therefore progestogens are required if HRT is prescribed in the usual fashion, to protect the endometrium from the effects of unopposed oestrogen.

D➤ 1. No   **1**

     2. No   **1**

     3. Yes   **1**

In validation, 45% of candidates have said it would be suitable to treat Mrs Peters with progestogens. This is hardly likely to work in the presence of 16-week fibroids.

The rest of this question is contentious as clinical practice can vary. Most surgeons would not attempt to remove a 16-week fibroid uterus vaginally. The whole concept of the laparoscopically assisted approach is to render difficult cases possible. By morcellation, a big mass may be brought out piecemeal through the vagina.

QUESTIONS

Score

Mrs Smith is 28 years of age and in her second pregnancy. She is aware of the recent publicity about 'home deliveries'. She asks you about the possibility of having a baby at home. In the discussion that ensues, she also asks whether DOMINO deliveries are available.

A➤ What is a DOMINO (domestic in and out) delivery?

B➤ In counselling the patient, list three potential benefits of a home confinement.

1.

2.

3.

C➤ List five relative contraindications to recommending a home confinement when counselling a patient at booking.

1.

2.

3.

4.

5.

ANSWERS/COMMENTS

Score

A➤ Where the same midwife sees the patient in the community setting and is subsequently available to deliver the baby in the hospital maternity unit.

2

The key points are continuity of midwife care, delivery in hospital and early discharge, usually six hours after delivery. Many candidates mentioned discharge within six hours, but failed to stress the continuity of the midwife involved.

B➤ 1. Familiar surroundings

1

2. Lower perinatal mortality rate

1

3. Children and family in close attendance

1

While cheaper (suggested by a number of candidates), in truth this is hardly a potential benefit one would discuss.

C➤ Any five of the following:

5

1. Primigravida
2. Multigravida over 35 years and parity >4
3. Poor home conditions
4. Poor obstetric history, including stillbirth and neonatal death
5. Previous low birth weight infant
6. Medical conditions such as diabetes or heart disease
7. Previous uterine surgery
8. Short stature or small shoe size, a rough guide to cephalopelvic disproportion

Antepartum haemorrhage, placenta praevia, pregnancy-induced hypertension and malpresentation are not acceptable. These are not apparent at the initial 'booking' of the patient but develop subsequently.

 Tip: Read the question.

Primigravida and short stature will not be considered as contraindications by many.

In one examination, candidates suggested 'GP unwilling and inexperienced'. This is not acceptable; a GP is not required. A midwife can undertake a home delivery on her own. She is an independent practitioner.

REST STATION

INTERACTIVE STATION

Score

Instructions to actress

You are Paula, a 22 year old, and you present to your GP surgery very tearful. You have been the victim of a rape after a party eight weeks previously and you have been too frightened to tell anyone until now. You have been feeling generally unwell, have missed two periods and have experienced frequency and breast tenderness. You suspect you may be pregnant.

You have performed a pregnancy test and the result is positive.

You are attending today to request a termination of pregnancy. Naturally you will enquire about complications. Having 'opened up' at last, you become increasingly agitated and upset as the interview continues, reflecting your own anger about the rape and distress of not coming forward previously.

You will eventually calm down and listen to the GP but only with some prompting.

Instructions to candidate

Paula is 22 years old and attends your surgery claiming rape. She has had a positive pregnancy test and wants a termination of pregnancy. She is very upset.

You are asked to conduct the consultation as if you are in your own surgery.

Please counsel Paula *fully*, offering what advice and support you deem necessary.

Instructions to examiner

At this station you are interested particularly in the candidate's ability to be kindly and supportive but firm. A candidate who allows the role player to take over the interview and swamp her/him with her rising hysteria has not done well. The candidate must be able to calm the 'victim' to allow necessary counselling and consultation to take place. Otherwise, the candidate will not have fulfilled his/her obligation. A relative or friend could offer a sympathetic ear. Four key areas should be covered: the risks of surgery, counselling support, screening the genitourinary tract and the patient's attitude to police involvement.

ANSWERS/COMMENTS

	Score
Scoring by the actress	
Appropriate eye contact	1
Listened attentively	1
Confidence in candidate	1
I would like to see this person again	1
Scoring by the examiner	
Main risks of abortion by surgical intervention:	1
infection, haemorrhage	
small risk of perforation	
small risk of infertility	
Screening for sexually transmitted diseases offered	1
Obtaining ongoing support and psychological counselling (e.g. Rape Crisis)	1
Police involvement discussed	1
Facilitator role successfully adopted (i.e. patient enabled to make own decision)	1
Interview time structured appropriately	1

This was another station which has resulted in quite a wide range of response from candidates. Range of marks scored by candidates out of ten: 4–10. Mean 7.5; standard deviation 2.5.

Some candidates voiced concern that this station disadvantaged conscientious objectors who were not prepared to be involved with termination of pregnancy. Whilst no station would require in-depth knowledge of the mechanism of termination of pregnancy, it is perfectly reasonable to expect candidates to have a working knowledge of the possible complications and risks involved with the procedure. At least, a clinican will need a sufficient understanding of the procedure to be able to counsel or manage an emergency situation effectively.

This station has been designed to test interactive communication skills and knowledge. The candidates need to demonstrate quite subtle interactive skills – sympathy and support but at the same time taking firm but gentle control of the conversation. They must demonstrate knowledge of the complications of a termination of pregnancy and the counselling and

ANSWERS/COMMENTS

Score

support required for a rape victim. One candidate scored very highly indeed by offering a termination in a different area to prevent any possibility of the rape victim meeting acquaintances at the local district hospital which might cause embarrassment.

Some candidates have demonstrated their knowledge and covered all the areas required of them but have done so in a brusque businesslike manner, adopting a very matter-of-fact approach.

One or two candidates demonstrated considerable sympathy and paid special attention to the psychological state of the patient but ran out of time before all essential aspects of the case had been discussed. It is this very fine balance that a good clinician must be able to demonstrate in the work setting.

QUESTIONS

A 35-year-old mother attends your surgery at 16 weeks' gestation. Her previous pregnancy was terminated at 20 weeks because spina bifida was detected.

A► From the above information, what is her risk of having another foetus affected by a neural tube defect?

Her serum α-fetoprotein was assayed the week before this clinic and returned as serum AFP >2.5 multiples of the median (MOM).

B► What is the significance of this result?

C► Would you offer to perform:

1. triple test?

   Yes/No

2. maternal chromosomal analysis?

   Yes/No

3. a foetal cordocentesis?

   Yes/No

4. detailed anomaly scan?

   Yes/No

5. chorionic villus sampling?

   Yes/No

D► List three conditions that will give a raised serum α-fetoprotein, excluding neural tube defect.

1.

2.

3.

ANSWERS/COMMENTS

	Score

A➤ 1%   1

In validation this question was very badly answered. Many candidates gave the risk of having a Down baby at 35 years of age despite the question clearly asking about the risk of a neural tube defect.

B➤ High level, further increases her risk   1

The question was based on the potential confusion between Down screening and screening for neural tube defect. Down syndrome results in a lower than normal fetoprotein result.

C➤ 1. No   1
     2. No   1
     3. No   1
     4. Yes   1
     5. No   1

Only a detailed ultrasound will detect spina bifida; indeed, most obstetricians would not perform an AFP assay. The triple test seeks to provide a more specific risk estimate of Down syndrome based on the composite screening of four variables: maternal age, maternal serum α-fetoprotein, maternal serum unconjugated oestriol and maternal serum human chorionic gonadotrophin. The question has already shown an increased risk of neural tube defect from the patient's family history and from a raised α-fetoprotein level. Although some 35-year-olds do ask for a triple test as an estimate of their risk for Down syndrome, it is not releveant in this context, which is screening for neural tube defects for an at-risk case.

Equally, maternal chromosomal analysis to check for balanced translocation and cordocentesis, to provide a sample of foetal blood for chromosomal analysis, are more relevant to Down screening. Chorionic villus sampling allows DNA probing and tissue cell culture to assess chromosomal distribution for Down syndrome.

ANSWERS/COMMENTS

Score
3

D► Any three of the following:

1. Posterior urethral valves in male foetus
2. Maternal liver disease
3. Preceding intrauterine growth retardation (IUGR)/pregnancy induced hypertension (PIH)/foetal death in some cases
4. Exomphalos
5. Twins
6. Congenital nephrosis
7. Turner syndrome
8. Trisomy 13

Wrong dates are not acceptable.

There is a long list of possible answers so that it should not be difficult to gain two or three marks here.

Raised α-fetoprotein at 16 weeks' gestation may be associated with problems later in the pregnancy (see answer D.3). The exact mechanism is unclear. However, the association is not strong enough to use as a screening test.

QUESTIONS

A➤ Explain how a mother would use a foetal movement chart.

B➤ 1. When would a mother in her first pregnancy first expect to feel movements?

2. When would a mother in her fourth pregnancy first expect to feel movements?

C➤ Classically, at what stage during gestation would you ask a mother to complete a foetal movement chart?

D➤ List four of the circumstances in which such a chart might be useful.

1.

2.

3.

4.

E➤ What trend would you observe as the pregnancy progresses?

ANSWERS/COMMENTS

Score

A► **The mother counts each time the baby kicks, starting at 9.00am. She stops counting when the baby has moved ten times. If she does not feel ten movements within 12 hours (i.e. by 9.00pm), she contacts the hospital.**
1 mark for ten kicks   **1**
1 mark for 12 hours   **1**

Candidates have to give the number of kicks and the time allowed to feel them to gain both marks.

B► 1. 20–22 weeks   **1**
    2. 16–18 weeks   **1**

In validation this was well answered.

Howlers! Three months; 28 weeks.

C► **32 weeks**   **1**

The original description of the Cardiff foetal movement chart proposed its use from 32 weeks' gestation. Many units in fact now use it any time after 28 weeks' gestation. Some obstetricians now query its usefulness at all.

D► **Any four of the following:**   **4**

    1. Diabetics
    2. Small-for-dates baby
    3. Pregnancy-induced hypertension
    4. Antepartum bleeding
    5. Postmaturity
    6. Maternal anxiety

Many candidates have listed 'anxiety' as an indication for using a foetal movement chart. Many feel this may increase anxiety but some will gain reassurance and the mother feels she is contributing to foetal surveillance.

ANSWERS/COMMENTS

Score

E▶ There is a gradual increase in the time it takes the mother to get ten kicks as the pregnancy advances towards term.

1

Many candidates have reported a gradual increase in movements until 38 weeks' gestation, when there was a sudden fall-off. In reality, although it takes longer to perceive ten discrete movements, a mother should still be able to count ten kicks within 12 hours, even at term. Failure to act on this may court tragedy.

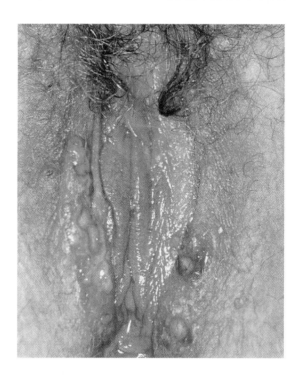

QUESTIONS

Score

A► Study the photograph.

1. What does it show?

2. What is the incubation period?

3. List three ways in which it may present (excluding ulceration).

   a

   b

   c

4. How is this condition diagnosed?

B► In gonorrhoea infections:

1. 5% of cases have a coinfection with *Trichomonas vaginalis*.

   True/False

2. A disseminated form can cause dermatitis.

   True/False

3. In penicillin-resistant strains the drug of choice is spectinomycin.

   True/False

4. Urethral swabs will be positive for gonorrhoea in the majority of cases.

   True/False

ANSWERS/COMMENTS

		Score
A▶	1. Herpes simplex, causing vulval ulceration and oedema	1
	2. 1–2 weeks	1
	3. Any three of the following:	3

3. Any three of the following:
    a Fever or flulike symptoms, preceding the onset of lesions in 30% of patients
    b Photophobia and severe headaches (mimicking viral meningitis) in 10% of cases
    c Dysuria
    d Acute urinary retention
    e In diabetics, severe ketoacidosis can occur within 12 hours of onset of infection

4. Either of the following: **1**
    a Viral culture of vesicular fluid
    b Electron microscopy of vesicular fluid
    Therefore, swabs should be taken *before* healing and crusting occur.

1. Almost 100% of candidates have identified the photograph correctly. It is in fact a very clear picture.

 Pitfall: *One candidate, however, tried to be too clever and gave an answer of HIV infection presenting as herpes labialis. It really does not pay to try to read too much into a question. If the answer seems obvious, it is probably because it is. Nevertheless, we have still had a smattering of syphilis, genital warts and gonorrhoea offered.*

2. Seventy percent of candidates have been correct here, but several gave an incubation period that was much too short (3–5 days) while others said as long as three weeks.

3. Many candidates have just redescribed the photograph, e.g. redness, swelling, vesicles, etc. The question was asking for alternative ways in which herpes may present. It does pay to stop and think before 'diving in' to answer a question. Generally, six minutes is sufficient to comfortably answer all OSCE stations. There is no need to rush. Obviously, the candidates who thought syphilis was the answer for part 1 were in trouble when trying to answer part 3. Approximately 20% mentioned urinary symptoms as a presentation.

ANSWERS/COMMENTS

	Score
B► 1. False	**1**
2. True	**1**
3. False	**1**
4. True	**1**

Almost 25% of candidates have answered all four parts correctly. The majority were correct for two out of four. Interestingly, part 1 has been answered incorrectly most often. There is in fact a 20–30% co-infection rate with *Trichomonas vaginalis*. Disseminated gonorrhoea can also cause arthritis which would have been an equally good stem for this question. Spectinomycin is not the drug of choice for penicillin-resistant strains; ciprofloxacin is. Urethral swabs would be positive in 70–90% of cases.

QUESTIONS

Mary attends your surgery early one Monday morning. She had unprotected intercourse at about 11.00pm on Saturday night. Her last menstrual period was about two weeks before. She is very upset because she does not want to be pregnant.

A► 1. What is the YUZPE regimen of postcoital contraception?

2. Please state the dose of each hormone used.

    a

    b

B► How long after unprotected intercourse may it be effectively used?

C► What is the failure rate?

D► Nausea and vomiting is the main side effect. What advice would you give to Mary if she vomited within one hour of the second dose?

E► An intrauterine contraceptive device may be used for postcoital contraception. Up to how long after unprotected intercourse may it be used?

F► At her three-week follow-up visit, Mary has not had a period. She used her YUZPE regimen correctly and has not had intercourse. Her pregnancy test is negative. She is keen to start the combined oral contraceptive pill. What would you do?

ANSWERS/COMMENTS

	Score

A► 1. A combination of ethinyloestradiol and levonorgestrel taken immediately and repeated 12 hours later   **1**

    2. a   100 µg ethinyloestradiol   **1**

       b   500 µg levonorgestrel   **1**

The majority of candidates succeeded with this question although some got confused with the amount of progestogen contained in the YUZPE regimen. Some candidates quoted the dose in each tablet rather than the total dose ingested on each occasion. Others did not mention how often the oestrogen and progestogen were to be taken.

B► 72 hours   **2**

All candidates have answered part B correctly.

C► 3–5% (mid-cycle)   **1**

A surprising number of candidates (approximately 55%) have felt that the failure rate for the YUZPE regimen was high, quoting up to 30%.

D► Repeat the dose and take an antiemetic.   **1**
or
Return to GP to discuss IUCD insertion.

Fifty percent have answered question D correctly.

E► Five days   **2**

Questions B and E are examples of 'weighted' scoring. The scores are higher for the correct answers because the information is fundamental.

ANSWERS/COMMENTS

Score

1

F➤ Give a progestogen (e.g. dydrogesterone 10 mg a day) for five days and start the pill on the second or third day of the withdrawal bleed.

or

Use barrier methods until next menses and start the combined oral contraceptive pill on the first day.

 Differentiator: *Several candidates have suggested incorrectly that the pregnancy test was repeated and then the contraceptive pill started on the first day of the next period. Examiners can only take the first answer even if the second part of that answer was correct. There is absolutely no point in repeating the pregnancy test if the stem has stated that her pregnancy test is negative. You are therefore to assume that Mary has not conceived.*

Approximately a third of candidates have been correct in stating that the contraceptive pill should be started on the first day of the next period. Only two thirds of these added that a barrier method must be used until then, which is an essential part of the answer. Surprisingly, no-one mentioned the possibility of offering a progestogen challenge test and commencing the pill on the second or third day of the induced withdrawal bleed.

QUESTIONS

A➤ For which four blood tests should a baby delivered to an Rh-negative mother have a blood sample taken from the umbilical cord at delivery?

1. _____

2. _____

3. _____

4. _____

B➤ What is a Kleihauer test?

_____

C➤ 1. On what day is the Guthrie test performed?

_____

2. Why is the Guthrie test performed?

a _____

b _____

D➤ 1. By which day should the umbilical stump usually separate?

_____

2. Should it be dressed?

Yes/No _____

ANSWERS/COMMENTS

	Score

A➤ Any four of the following: **4**

1. Blood group
2. Haemoglobin
3. Coombs test
4. Bilirubin test
5. Cord gases

During validation, 40% of candidates answered Kleihauer test. This test cannot be performed on foetal blood.

B➤ Measures the amount of foetal blood in the maternal circulation   **1**

It was unbelievable how many candidates have given the correct definition yet also included it as an answer for question A – read the question!

C➤ 1. Sixth day   **1**
    2. a To detect phenylketonuria   **1**
       b To detect hypothyroidism   **1**

Only 30% of candidates have given the correct answer to part 1. Most candidates knew what was being tested.

The Guthrie test is a heel prick sample, taken after the baby has had 48 hours of an adequate protein diet, whether breast or bottle fed. All babies should undergo screening for phenylketonuria and hypo-thyroidism, performed by measuring phenylalanine and thyroid-stimulating hormone levels respectively. Some units are also carrying out routine screening for cystic fibrosis as well as anonymous HIV antibody screening to assess the prevalence of this condition.

D➤ 1. 8–10 days   **1**
    2. No, it dries quicker if exposed to air.   **1**

Again, only 30% of candidates have given the correct answer for part 1. Most gave 3–5 days.

Howler! 30 days.

All candidates have given the correct answer for part 2.

QUESTIONS

Infant feeding is an important area of care.

A➤ List four important advantages associated with breast feeding.

1.

2.

3.

4.

B➤ If a mother who wishes to breast feed cannot do so initially because she has had general anaesthesia for delivery, what can be done?

C➤ Midwives should encourage the mother to breast feed at home. For how many days after delivery does the midwife usually call on the mother at home?

D➤ In a bottle fed baby at the end of the first week:

1. How much feed should the baby be taking in a 24-hour period?

2. How many feeds should the baby be receiving in a 24-hour period?

E➤ In what solution should you sterilize the bottles?

F➤ At what age should solids start?

ANSWERS/COMMENTS

	Score

A➤ Any four of the following: **4**

1. Contains protein, fat and solute content designed for babies
2. Promotes bonding
3. Reduces infection by providing passive immunity via maternal antibodies
4. Cheap
5. No risk of infection from bottles
6. Reduces atopy

In validation, most candidates scored two or three. Some candidates suggested that it caused less obesity. While we agree this is true, it is not considered an important advantage. Neither were the following novel suggestions:

Readily available on demand
No preparation required
It is the right temperature
'Instant fast food'

B➤ A 5% dextrose feed may be offered.   **1**

Ninety percent of candidates have suggested the use of a breast pump and expression. However, there will be no milk production at this stage. Even if milk was present, general anaesthesia is used in the emergency setting and it is unlikely that there would be time to express it.

C➤ Ten days   **1**

D➤ 1. 150 ml/kg/day   **1**
     2. Six feeds/24 hours   **1**

This section has been poorly answered with less than 50% correct answers.

E➤ Dilute hypochlorite solution   **1**

This is the type of information with which a well-informed GP should be able to help a mother. Again, this section has been poorly answered with only 50% of candidates giving the correct answer.

F➤ Around four months   **1**

A wide range of answers have been offered, ranging from six weeks to 18 months!

QUESTIONS

Score

Mrs Scott is 29 years old and presents with a history of superficial and deep dyspareunia since the birth of her last child eight months ago. This was a normal vaginal delivery, with a second-degree tear. She is bottle feeding, having fed on demand for three months. She has one other child, a hyperactive three-year-old.

A➤ List the two most likely causes for her superficial dyspareunia.

1. _____

2. _____

B➤ Outline three further questions you would wish to ask her in order to evaluate her symptom of deep dyspareunia.

1. _____

2. _____

3. _____

C➤ In assessing a likely cause for her deep dyspareunia, list two other questions you would ask.

1. _____

2. _____

D➤ When you examine Mrs Scott, list three features you would need to elicit or exclude to reach your final diagnosis (regarding deep dyspareunia).

1. _____

2. _____

3. _____

ANSWERS/COMMENTS

	Score

A► 1. Badly healed episiotomy scar   **1**

2. Vaginismus – tension/tiredness/depression   **1**

Most candidates did well here. The stem has included several clues. Mrs Scott had tried feeding on demand and given up. She has a hyperactive child. Tiredness and feelings of inability to cope account for a considerable amount of psychosexual dysfunction in the first year after delivery. The situation is often further strained by the partner feeling left out, redundant or jealous of the attention the child is receiving.

B► Any three of the following: **3**

1. Nature of pain
2. Does it stop when coitus stops or continue afterwards?
3. Is it positional?
4. How often does it occur?

This question asks the candidates to list basic questions you would ask to further *evaluate* the symptom of deep dyspareunia. This is really undergraduate knowledge yet in validation only 5% of candidates were correct. Many asked questions related to a general gynaecological history: when was the last cervical smear, what contraception was used, presence of discharge, etc.

 Tip: In the absence of a clinical or viva, examination of basic clinical skills can only be achieved in this way.

In the postgraduate examinations run by the Royal College of Anaesthetists, there are pass/fail questions, which you must get right to pass. The Royal College of Obstetricians and Gynaecologists does not currently have this type of question, but certainly a basic clinical station such as this one could legitimately be included as a pass/fail station.

ANSWERS/COMMENTS

Score

C➤ Any two of the following: 2

1. Did she have any puerperal infection, i.e. smelly lochia, retained products?
2. Does she have congestive dysmenorrhoea?
3. Explore psychogenic factors.

You are trying to exclude pelvic infection or endometriosis as causes. Vaginismus is more likely to contribute to *superficial* dyspareunia. Pelvic venous congestion can produce pain that continues after coitus ceases. The question is aimed at testing the candidate's ability to think laterally and look at causes other than those in the stem, i.e. episiotomy and stress.

D➤ Any three of the following: 3

1. Cervical excitation
2. Discharge
3. Adnexal masses
4. Tender and nodular uterosacral ligaments

The question asks for features you need to look for regarding *deep* dyspareunia, yet in validation, candidates listed narrow introitus, tender introitus and narrow vagina, all of which relate to *superficial* dyspareunia.

 Tip: Again, read the question!

QUESTIONS

Elizabeth is a 21-year-old insulin-dependent diabetic who presents for a repeat prescription of the combined oral contraceptive pill. Your practice nurse has suggested she sees you as she is thinking about stopping the pill and trying to have a baby.

Her blood results from her last diabetic clinic attendance are:

Glycosylated Hb	12% (5.6–7.6)
Cholesterol	6.2 mmol/l (4.0–6.5)
Creatinine	67 mmol/l (45–125)
Random glucose	11 mmol/l (3.2–11.1)

A➤ What immediate advice would you give this patient in response to her wish to become pregnant?

B➤ Which three members of the extended primary health care team have an important role in managing this patient's future pregnancy?

1.

2.

3.

C➤ Give three maternal complications of diabetes in pregnancy.

1.

2.

3.

QUESTIONS

D➤ Give three foetal complications of diabetes in pregnancy.

1. _____

2. _____

3. _____

ANSWERS/COMMENTS

	Score

A➤ Improve her diabetic control.

1

This question was specifically related to preconception counselling in an insulin-dependent diabetic.

 *Differentiator: Many candidates have suggested that folic acid should be started immediately. Really, this is not relevant until Elizabeth is ready to try to conceive and clearly she should not try to conceive until her diabetic control is considerably better. Folic acid would be the next step once good diabetic control had been achieved and obviously is most beneficial if it is already being taken at the time of conception and throughout organogenesis. The current recommendations are 400 μg a day to prevent **occurrence** and 5 mg a day to prevent **recurrence** of neural tube defects.*

B➤ Any three of the following:

3

1. Diabetic liaison nurse
2. Community midwife
3. Health visitor
4. GP
5. Dietician

It was surprising how many candidates offered obstetrician or paediatrician as an answer to this question. The stem clearly asked for three members of the extended primary health care team. The extended primary health care team (PHCT) are those working in the practice and those who visit the practice and/or patients in the community. Almost 25% of candidates offered dietician as an answer. Originally we had not included this in our answer pool as in many areas dieticians are attached solely to hospitals, but that is not the case in every area and there are some community-based dieticians or those that rotate through primary health care clinics, even if the central base is within the hospital. We have therefore added this to our pool of answers. There was also some debate as to whether a general practitioner was a member of the extended primary health care team but he or she is really a member of the core primary health care team.

ANSWERS/COMMENTS

Score

C➤ Any three of the following: 3

1. Poor diabetic control/increased insulin resistance
2. Infections – thrush, urinary tract infection
3. Pregnancy-induced hypertension
4. Accelerated diabetic complications – retinopathy, nephropathy
5. Maternal soft tissue injury/birth trauma
6. Polyhydramnios

Only 16% of candidates were completely correct; 30% of candidates offered preterm labour as a maternal complication of diabetes and pregnancy. This is not a *specific* problem of diabetes though it may occur secondary to polyhydramnios.

D➤ Any three of the following: 3

1. Increased foetal anomalies
2. Macrosomia
3. Hypoglycaemia
4. Respiratory distress syndrome
5. Jaundice
6. Polycythaemia
7. Preterm labour (secondary to polyhydramnios)
8. Birth trauma
9. Intrauterine death

The majority gave very good answers here although some candidates listed three different types of foetal abnormality. We felt that that was inappropriate. We have a list of nine possible answers so it is not difficult to collect points on this question, and we felt that candidates should offer three different types of complications rather than three examples of one type of complication. Remember that all abnormalities are more common with diabetes, while sacral agenesis is *specific* to poor control.

119

QUESTIONS

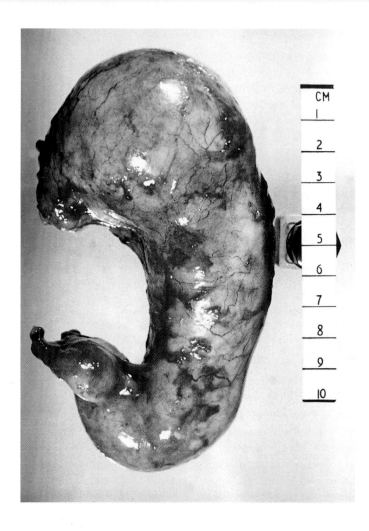

QUESTIONS

A➤ Study the photograph. What does it show?

_____

B➤ List three clinical features that a patient with this condition might complain of.

1. _____

2. _____

3. _____

C➤ Define chronic pelvic pain (CPP).

_____

D➤ In CPP:

1. In approximately 70% of women there is no identifiable pathology.

    True/False _____

2. Medroxyprogesterone acetate alone is ineffective therapy.

    True/False _____

3. Pelvic venous congestion often presents with postcoital pain.

    True/False _____

4. There is an association between CPP and childhood sexual abuse.

    True/False _____

5. Pelvic venous congestion is common in the postmenopausal years.

    True/False _____

ANSWERS/COMMENTS

Score

A➤ Hydrosalpinx

1

We have been rather surprised that only 50% of candidates correctly identified a hydrosalpinx. The photograph is very clear. One candidate suggested that it showed an ectopic pregnancy but this would have been a very large tubal pregnancy indeed and would have most certainly ruptured before reaching this size.

 Howlers! *Enlarged uterus with fibroids or ovarian cyst. Other candidates have suggested an appendix!*

B➤ Any three of the following:

3

1. Heavy, irregular menses
2. Dysmenorrhoea
3. Dyspareunia
4. Chronic pelvic pain
5. Infertility

Hydrosalpinx or pyosalpinx are usually manifestations of chronic pelvic inflammatory disease. Patients may present with acute or chronic manifestations but in asking for a list of three clinical features of a patient with a hydrosalpinx, we had rather hoped for a symptom related to chronic infection.

Those candidates who have offered temperature, vaginal discharge and acute abdominal pain, which are acute manifestations of pelvic infection, were incorrect. Some candidates have suggested 'palpable mass' as a clinical feature of which this patient might complain. This would assume that the patient was able to palpate the mass abdominally, which would mean that it must be at least as large as a 12- or 14-week gravid uterus. This is most unlikely. Whilst a painful inflammatory mass can develop when bowel and omentum are stuck around a pyosalpinx, this mass is normally only palpable on bimanual assessment.

C➤ Chronic pelvic pain is pain located in the pelvis which has been present for at least six months.

1

 Differentiator: *The definition of chronic pelvic pain has caused some problems, with less than 20% of candidates offering a correct answer. Most candidates have glibly suggested it was pain confined to the pelvis but have not defined the length of time over which the pain occurred. Others have suggested that pain would have had to be present for one year and some for only three months.*

ANSWERS/COMMENTS

	Score
D➤ 1. True	1
2. False	1
3. True	1
4. True	1
5. False	1

1. Chronic pain accounts for 30% of gynaecological referrals. In 60–75% of these women, there is no identifiable pathology.

2. Most CPP is thought to be due to pelvic venous congestion and/or psychological causes. Medroxyprogesterone acetate 50 mg a day is very effective during treatment but relapses occur after cessation. It cannot be said to be ineffective. However, medroxyprogesterone acetate and psychotherapy together may achieve sustained relief.

3. Two thirds of women with pelvic venous congestion suffer pain after intercourse with many consumed with pain for up to an hour afterwards.

4. There is a 30% incidence of childhood sexual abuse in CPP sufferers. However, the aetiology of CPP is multifactorial. The role of psychological factors has been debated for some time and childhood sexual abuse may not be a specific aetiological factor. The key word in the question is 'association'.

5. Pelvic venous congestion is never seen in women who are older than 60 years of age and in a recent study the median age for such patients was 30 years.

QUESTIONS

A couple are attending the surgery for the results of their infertility investigations. The female's hormone profile is as follows:

Prolactin	300 (150–500) iu/l
Thyroid-stimulating hormone	2.08 u/l (1.8–13.4)
Free T4	14.9 pmol/l (9.0–27.0)
LH	9 milliIu/ml (1.8–13.4)
FSH	5 milliIu/ml (3.0–12.0)
Luteal phase progesterones	7 ng/ml, 12 ng/ml, 9 ng/ml
Rubella	Immune

The male partner's semen analysis is as follows:

Volume	2 ml
Total count	86 million/ml
Motility	60%
Abnormal forms	20%
Mar test	Negative

You decide to treat the couple in a primary care setting.

QUESTIONS

Score

A► What is the main reason this lady has failed to achieve pregnancy?

B► 1. What would be your first-line therapy?

2. Quote the usual starting regimen.

3. In counselling a patient commencing this therapy:

   a There is a known association with ovarian cancer.

   True/False

   b It should not be prescribed in the presence of an unfavourable postcoital test.

   True/False

   c The multiple pregnancy rate is trebled.

   True/False

   d Hyperstimulation syndrome is a recognized complication.

   True/False

C► What two other baseline investigations would be justified for you to organize from your surgery to investigate this couple?

1.

2.

D► What is a Mar test?

ANSWERS/COMMENTS

	Score

A➤ Anovulation

Score: 1

The three luteal phase progesterones are low, indicating anovulation.

B➤ 1. Clomiphene citrate
2. 50 mg per day from day 2 to 6 of her cycle
3. a True
   b True
   c False
   d True

Score: 1, 1, 1, 1, 1, 1

Most candidates have answered clomiphene citrate correctly. Many gave the correct dose but omitted the days of the cycle on which it should be given.

 Differentiator: *Only 10% of candidates got all four parts of B.3 correct. Clomiphene citrate can lead to cervical hostility, therefore you would not prescribe it for a woman with a negative postcoital test. Clomiphene citrate can in a small number of cases lead to hyperstimulation. It does, so far, less often than other fertility treatment, but hyperstimulation remains a **recognized** complication. The multiple pregnancy rate is one in 70.*

C➤ 1. Hysterosalpingogram
2. Postcoital test

Score: 1, 1

During validation, candidates were unhappy with hysterosalpingogram, which they considered was a hospital investigation, but it can be ordered in the same way as a barium enema direct from the surgery. The postcoital test should have come to mind as it appeared in question B.3b. Follicle tracking to monitor ovulation, suggested by a few candidates, is not considered a baseline investigation.

 Howlers!
1. *Day 21 progesterone – already done.*
2. *Antisperm antibodies – not with a normal semen analysis.*
3. *Serum, testosterone and sex hormone-binding globulin – not helpful. They may be useful to investigate a case of polycystic ovarian syndrome (one cause of anovulation) but the question asked for 'baseline' investigations for this couple. In this case the FSH:LH ratio does not indicate PCO.*

D➤ A test of sperm antibodies

Score: 1

 Differentiator: *Poorly answered. Many said it was a postcoital test.*

REST STATION

STRUCTURED ORAL

Instructions to candidate

Mrs Khan, an accountant, is currently 17 weeks into her first pregnancy. She booked at 14 weeks. Recently, she was contacted by the antenatal clinic sister at the local hospital and asked to reattend to discuss some results. The sister explained she could not discuss results over the telephone.

Owing to her mother's recent illness, Mrs Khan requested that the results should be faxed through to your surgery so she could attend for discussion, as this was a much easier journey for her.

Study the following results:

> TPHA
> Positive to dilutions of 1:8
>
> VDRL
> Positive to dilutions of 1:16

The examiner will discuss the case with you.

Instructions to examiner

A► What do these test results mean? (fill in mark 1 on candidate's mark sheet).

Answer should be _____

B► How is the treponemal haemagglutination test (TPHA) performed? (fill in mark 2 on candidate's mark sheet).

Answer should be _____

C► Name three situations in which biological false-positive results can occur (fill in marks 3, 4 and 5 on candidate's mark sheet).

1. _____

2. _____

3. _____

STRUCTURED ORAL

Score

D➤ Why is it still important to screen for syphilis? (fill in mark 6 on candidate's mark sheet).

Answer should be _____

E➤ Name two characteristics of congenital syphilis (fill in marks 7 and 8 on candidate's mark sheet).

1. _____

2. _____

F➤ Name two tests that are more reliable than either VDRL or TPHA (fill in marks 9 and 10 on candidate's mark sheet).

1. _____

2. _____

ANSWERS/COMMENTS

	Score

A➤ These results are weakly positive. — **1**

 Differentiator: This station was very poorly answered.

Range of marks scored by candidates during validation was 1–8; mean 3.1, standard deviation 1.68.

Again, it can be argued that this is a standard antenatal booking test and as such it represents basic core knowledge.

B➤ The TPHA test detects reagin, an antibody-like substance produced early in treponemal infection and some other conditions, i.e. non-specific test. — **1**

C➤ Any three of the following: — **3**

1. Malaria
2. Leprosy
3. Glandular fever
4. Pregnancy
5. Acute stages of several viral infections

Several candidates offered yaws or pinta as answers. Athough these are examples of false positives they are *not* examples of biological false positives as yaws and pinta are also treponemal infections.

D➤ Though less common than previously, maternal syphilis is still screened for because it can cause congenital syphilis in the infant. Treatment before 16 weeks' gestation can prevent this. — **1**

ANSWERS/COMMENTS

	Score

E➤ Any two of the following: **2**

1. Parrot's nodes
2. Frontal bossing
3. 'Hot cross bun' skull
4. High-arched palate
5. Hutchinson's teeth
6. The triad of interstitial keratitis, Hutchinson's teeth and eighth nerve deafness is pathognomonic.

Several candidates have suggested sabre tibia as an answer. This is a characteristic of tertiary syphilis, not of congenital syphilis.

This station can be restructured as an interactive station with a very irate Mrs Khan feeling personally insulted by the perceived insinuation that she had syphilis. This would be designed to test the tact and diplomacy of candidates and their understanding of the limitation of the test. Structured orals, of course, test factual knowledge more than interactive skills.

F➤ 1. Fluorescent treponemal antibody absorbed test (FTA). Very sensitive and positive in primary syphilis. **1**

2. Treponemal pallidum immobilization test (TPI). More specific. Remains negative with the secondary stage. **1**

QUESTIONS

You receive a discharge summary about a 46-year-old patient who had a total abdominal hysterectomy and bilateral salpingo-oophorectomy two weeks previously for heavy periods. Her histology report reads:

The uterus is enlarged, measuring 10 cm × 6 cm. The myometrium shows evidence of adenomyosis. The endometrium is 15 mm in depth and microscopically has the appearance of cystic glandular hyperplasia.

The cervix shows evidence of CIN1 which is completely excised. The left ovary is normal. The right ovary contains a 5 cm endometriotic cyst.

A➤ Define adenomyosis.

B➤ Define cystic glandular hyperplasia.

C➤ This patient should:

1. be advised to have a vault smear in six months.

   Yes/No

2. be advised never to have hormone replacement therapy.

   Yes/No

3. be commenced on Prempak-C (conjugated oestrogens 625 μg, norgesterol 150 μg) 1.25 mg.

   Yes/No

4. have yearly CA125 in view of the risk of recurrent endometrioid ovarian carcinoma.

   Yes/No

5. have a serum oestradiol level performed.

   Yes/No

QUESTIONS

Score

D➤ Give three non-gynaecological presentations of endometriosis.

1. _____

2. _____

3. _____

ANSWERS/COMMENTS

Score

A➤ Adenomyosis occurs when the endometrial glands invade the myometrium. Sections of the uterus show a thickened myometrium with dark spots which are areas of endometrium and retained menstrual blood.

1

The majority of candidates have given a correct definition of adenomyosis. One or two have confused adenomyosis with cystic glandular hyperplasia and have given a definition for question B to question A.

 Howler! *Benign enlargement of the myometrium – this would be an adequate description for a fibroid but this is not adenomyosis.*

B➤ Cystic glandular hyperplasia is a proliferative area of growth of the endometrium due to anovulation and persistent unopposed exposure to oestrogen.

1

 Differentiator: *Many people have described proliferative growth of the endometrium but did not complete the definition by alluding to the association with anovulation and persistent unopposed exposure to oestrogen, and we felt that this was a vital part of the definition.*

 Pitfall: *Several candidates have thought that cystic glandular hyperplasia was a premalignant condition. They had obviously confused it with hyperplasia involving architectural atypia which is an unstable cellular change. Sadly, surprisingly few candidates have got the definition entirely correct.*

C➤ 1. No

    2. No

    3. No

    4. No

    5. No

1
1
1
1
1

Almost a third of the candidates have given entirely correct answers to all five parts to this question. Where candidates most commonly went wrong were with parts 1 and 4. Since both adenomyosis and cystic glandular hyperplasia are benign conditions there is absolutely no point in performing a vault smear following surgery. A vault smear is only performed in cases where the indication for hysterectomy is carcinoma of the cervix or uterus though some are of the opinion it is of little value even in these cases. There was CIN1 present but it was completely excised. There is also no point in performing annual CA125 estimations. CA125 is a tumour marker for certain types of squamous ovarian cancer. There was no evidence of

ANSWERS/COMMENTS

ovarian tumour in this case, only endometriosis. There is no association between ovarian endometrioid cancer and cystic glandular hyperplasia. Adenomyosis has been put in here to confuse the issue. There is an association between pelvic endometriosis and endometrial tumours.

Some candidates have felt that this patient should have been commenced on Kliofem, a continuous combined preparation containing 2 mg 17β oestradiol with 1 mg norethisterone. This is controversial. Since the patient has had a hysterectomy there is no indication for prescribing progestogens to combat the effects of unopposed oestrogen on the endometrium. However, there may be a theoretical benefit in continuing with progestogens if the patient had marked osteoporosis. Norethisterone has a direct effect on bone density in its own right. This, however, is rather 'small print' for a DRCOG examination question. Moreover, the stem does not contain information to suggest that either of these indications is pertinent here. The stem *does* indicate evidence of pelvic endometriosis, however, in mentioning a 5 cm endometriotic cyst. Many authorities would suggest allowing six months to elapse before commencing hormone replacement therapy to avoid any endometriotic recurrence. Others would start HRT straight away but recommend a continuous combined preparation to suppress microscopic deposits.

D➤ Any three of the following:

3

1. Rectal bleeding
2. Haematuria
3. Obstruction of ureter or bowel
4. Haemoptosis
5. Menstrual epilepsy

This question asked for three non-gynaecological presentations of endometriosis; it is incorrect to offer deposits/bleeding in an episiotomy scar or subumbilical laparoscopy scar.

QUESTIONS

Score

You are the gynaecology SHO on call when a 26-year-old lady is admitted to casualty complaining of irregular brown discharge and some lower abdominal pains. Her last proper period was five weeks ago. She has been actively trying to conceive. In the past she has had a termination of pregnancy at eight weeks' gestation. The pregnancy test is positive.

Answer the following questions regarding management.

A▶ What would you consider to be the two most likely differential diagnoses in this case?

1. _____

2. _____

B▶ When you are examining the patient what signs might you look for to help distinguish between them (name two)?

1. _____

2. _____

C▶ What test would you organize to assist diagnosis if there is still doubt after examination?

_____

D▶ Describe three features you would be looking for on this test that might distinguish between the possible diagnoses.

1. _____

2. _____

3. _____

E▶ If the results of the test are equivocal what would be your next steps in management (list two)?

1. _____

2. _____

ANSWERS/COMMENTS

	Score

A➤ 1. Ectopic pregnancy   1
    2. Threatened miscarriage   1

B➤ Any two of the following: 2

1. Cervical excitation
2. Softening of the cervical os
3. Os open
4. Forniceal tenderness and/or fullness

This was well done. Everyone was aware of the two differential diagnoses and most candidates offered cervical excitation and forniceal tenderness as the two clinical signs they would look for to help distinguish between them.

One or two candidates commented on blood loss. It is commonly believed that if the loss is heavy this indicates an intrauterine pregnancy and that ectopic pregnancies produce a light, intermittent loss or brownish discharge. Actually, this can be misleading. A cornual ectopic pregnancy can rupture into the uterine cavity and cause profuse loss.

In this particular example, blood loss is not relevant anyway. The question clearly asked what signs would be useful to distinguish between the two possible diagnoses in 'the patient'. The stem refers only to irregular brown discharge.

Similarly, passage of products of conception is irrelevant to this scenario. Again, in general, this can be a clinical pitfall. Ectopic pregnancies produce β-hCG and stimulate a decidual reaction in the endometrium. Shedding and passage of a decidual cast can, to the naked eye, be mistaken for products.

C➤ Pelvic ultrasound   1

Everyone gave ultrasound as the test needed to assist diagnosis. Fifty percent of candidates were more specific and requested transvaginal ultrasonography which does provide better resolution.

D➤ 1. Intrauterine sac, possibly foetal poles/pseudogestational sac   1
    2. Complex adnexal cyst   1
    3. Free fluid in the pouch of Douglas   1

ANSWERS/COMMENTS

E➤ Any two of the following:

1. If abdominal probe scan performed, consider repeating with vaginal probe for better resolution.
2. Repeat scan in one week's time if no further deterioration of symptoms.
3. Perform quantitative serial serum β-hCG and repeat ultrasound if steady rise.

Most candidates were comfortable with the features they would look for on ultrasound to confirm the diagnosis of ectopic. However, very few candidates had a sound grasp of the logical steps of management if the scan result was equivocal. Most wished to proceed straight to laparoscopy.

QUESTIONS

Score

Perinatal mortality is still used as the main crude measure of antenatal care. It has fallen dramatically over the last 40 years.

A➤ Define perinatal mortality.

B➤ List five principal causes of perinatal mortality.

1.
2.
3.
4.
5.

C➤ 1. What is the average perinatal mortality for units in the UK?

2. List two drug interventions directly contributing to the reduction in this rate in the last ten years.

a

b

D➤ Is perinatal mortality greater in a hospital unit or a GP unit?

ANSWERS/COMMENTS

	Score

A► **Perinatal mortality rates comprise all stillbirths after 24 weeks' gestation and all first-week neonatal deaths per 1000 total births.**

Score: **1**

When validating this station, only one candidate answered this question correctly. There are three key points in the definition:

1. Still births after 24 weeks
2. First-week neonatal deaths
3. Per 1000 total births.

Many variations have been offered.

B► **Any five of the following:**

Score: **5**

1. Prematurity
2. Congenital abnormalities
3. Birth asphyxia
4. Birth trauma
5. Infection
6. Rhesus disease
7. Unexplained

Most candidates have achieved at least three correct answers. Meconium aspiration is included in birth asphyxia and is not accepted as a separate answer. Prematurity and respiratory distress syndrome will not be accepted as two separate answers as the former causes the latter. Either one would be accepted. Congenital malformations are more common in countries that do not allow therapeutic terminations.

ANSWERS/COMMENTS

	Score
C► 1. 8–10 per 1000	**1**
2. a Artificial lung surfactant	**1**
b Use of steroids	**1**

1. Sixty-five percent of candidates gave the correct answer. Those who were incorrect were usually too optimistic, giving rates of 1–2 per 1000.
2. Tocolytics, suggested by 40% of candidates, have not made a major impact in reducing the number of babies who deliver preterm, which is the major cause of mortality. Some candidates argued that the use of tocolytics delayed delivery long enough to transfer in utero to a better neonatal unit. This is too tenuous an argument. Antibiotics, of course, made their impact more than 20 years ago.

 Tip: Answer the question directly; do not make several chess moves!

 Howler! Folic acid.

D► Hospital unit   **1**

In general, only low-risk pregnancies are booked to deliver in a GP unit, therefore the perinatal mortality will be lower.

141

Circuit C

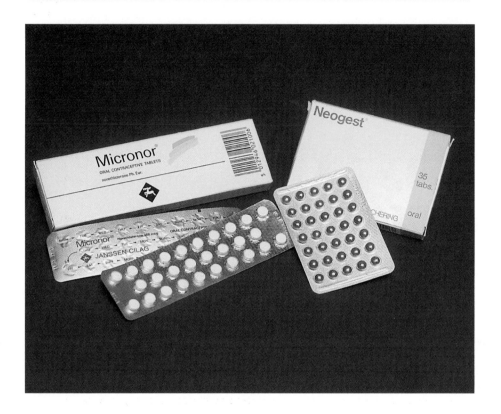

QUESTIONS

Study the packets of contraceptive pills in front of you.

A➤ Name two mechanisms of their contraceptive action.

1.

2.

B➤ List three categories of women for which this would be an especially useful form of contraception.

1.

2.

3.

C➤ Irregular bleeding can occur in:

5% of users
10% of users
30% of users
50% of users

Give one answer

D➤ Give one feature of a woman's past gynaecological history which would make this form of contraception relatively strongly contra-indicated.

E➤ This form of contraception must be taken every day and:

1. at the same time every day.

   Yes/No

2. within one hour of the same time every day.

   Yes/No

3. within three hours of the same time every day.

   Yes/No

ANSWERS/COMMENTS

Score

A▶ 1. Cervical mucus changes (*MUST* have this answer)   **1**
And one of the following:
2. Ovulation is prevented or interrupted (in 60% of cases)   **1**
    or
3. Some antinidatory action on the endometrium (atrophic endometrium)

In validation all candidates mentioned cervical mucus hostility and 50% commented on reduction in ovulation; 50% mentioned the antinidatory effect. Suppression of ovulation here is insufficient. This is an example of a weighted answer and cervical mucus changes must be mentioned. Several candidates mentioned reduction in tubular motility but this is *not* a contraceptive function. Currently only 6% of pill users take the 'mini-pill'.

B▶ Any three of the following: **3**

1. Older women, especially smokers over the age of 35 years
2. Breastfeeding women
3. Women who suffer side effects with the combined contraceptive pill
4. Medical conditions that are contraindications to combined contraceptive pill
5. Migraine sufferers
6. Sickle cell disease (homozygous)

 Howlers! Many candidates mentioned that this was a suitable method of contraception for those with irregular cycles. At least 30% of women on progestogen-only pills have irregular bleeding. Some become amenorrhoeic. Others stated it would be good contraception in those cases where contraception did not need to be 'desperately maximal'!

Some candidates considered it to be suitable only for non-smokers under the age of 35 – a complete reversal of the truth. Generally, this question has been answered badly. The failure rate of the progestogen-only pill is relatively high in under-25-year-olds (over 3/100 woman-years).

C▶ 50%   **1**

 Differentiator: In validation, this question was very poorly answered – only 10% of candidates gave the correct answer.

ANSWERS/COMMENTS

	Score

D➤ Previous ectopic pregnancy
or
Previous symptomatic functional cysts

Score: **1**

 Howler! Pregnancy! It is, of course, smokers, breastfeeding women and those with a thrombogenic risk that we **recommend** take the progestogen-only pill. Only 30% have been correct.

It is worth mentioning that there may be a link between increased body weight (over 80 kg) and failure rate, similar to the progestogen-secreting vaginal ring. Some experts suggest that overweight women take two progestogen-only pills per day.

E➤ Within three hours of the same time each day, therefore:

1. No   **1**
2. No   **1**
3. Yes   **1**

Generally, two out of the three answers were correct.

QUESTIONS

Score

Your patient is a 20-year-old single parent, having had two previous miscarriages by different partners. The membranes ruptured at 26 weeks and she is now beginning to contract.

Study the accompanying ultrasound report:

> There is gross oligohydramnios, with only small pools of liquor measuring 1.3 mm and 1.6 mm across. The walls of the uterus hug the foetus and make measurement of the abdominal circumference impossible. The foetus is in breech presentation, legs extended, biparietal diameter is 67.5 mm and estimated foetal weight is 600 g.

A► 1. What is the percentage survival rate at 26 weeks?

2. What percentage of survivors at this gestation have long-term morbidity?

3. Name two long-term problems often encountered by survivors?

   a

   b

B► Name a potential additional non-infective complication in this case.

QUESTIONS

Score

C➤ How would you manage this case?

1. Use tocolytics to halt labour.

   Yes/No
   _____

2. Use indomethacin to halt labour.

   Yes/No
   _____

3. Allow vaginal breech delivery.

   Yes/No
   _____

4. Deliver by caesarean section.

   Yes/No
   _____

D➤ In a maximum of two sentences, state the reason for your decision.

   _____

   _____

ANSWERS/COMMENTS

	Score

A▸ 1. 50–60% — 1

2. 70–80% — 1

3. Any two of the following: — 2
   a Short stature
   b Low IQ
   c Cerebral palsy
   d Developmental delay
   e Chronic respiratory disease (bronchopulmonary dysplasia)
   f Retinopathy of prematurity

In validation, answers from parts 1 and 2 varied widely from 5% to 90%. Only a third of candidates provided the correct ranges. With a total of six acceptable answers for part 3, this section should be easy.

 Howler! A.3 – *Single parent may lack support.*

B▸ Pulmonary hypoplasia — 1
or
Limb contractures

This is obviously alluding to the gross oligohydramnios in this case which will predispose to limb contractures and pulmonary hypoplasia as there is no room for foetal movement in utero. It is obviously important to read the stem very carefully, particularly when there is a detailed ultrasound report provided.

C▸ 1. No — 1

2. No — 1

3. Yes — 1

4. No — 1

Answers to ethical issues are always difficult to give as a simple yes or no. Nevertheless, in this context one must remember that this is a single parent who is only 20 years old and that she has already had two previous partners. To scar her uterus for an infant with such a small chance of survival is probably not justified, particularly if the current relationship may be unstable.

ANSWERS/COMMENTS

Score

D➤ The outlook for foetal survival is appalling. She is young and single – why scar her womb?

1

Obviously, candidates' attitudes to question C were reiterated in their answers to D. Many understood the reasons for avoiding the caesarean section; others wanted to deliver by caesarean to maximize foetal chances.

QUESTIONS

Study the following traces, A–E on pages 153 and 154.

A➤ 1. Which trace is most likely to be associated with the second stage?

2. What is the physiological mechanism for this?

B➤ 1. Which trace is most likely to be associated with a maternal pyrexia of 38.5°C?

2. List three tests you would perform in labour to assess the cause.

   a

   b

   c

C➤ 1. Which is the most sinister trace?

2. What does it represent?

3. What further test is indicated?

D➤ What interpretation would you put on variable decelerations?

QUESTIONS

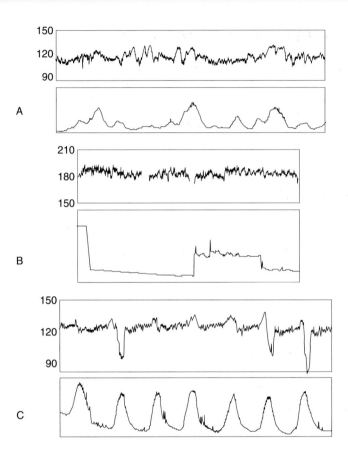

QUESTIONS

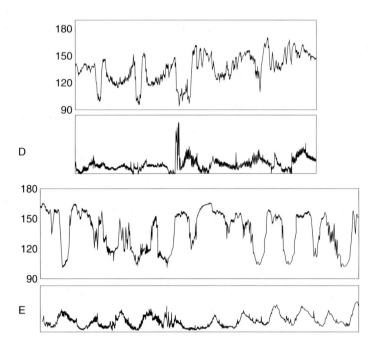

ANSWERS/COMMENTS

	Score

A➤ 1. Trace C (early deceleration with stable baseline and good beat-to-beat variability) — **1**

2. Head compression, e.g. during descent, is associated with a vasovagal reflex slowing of the heart — **1**

Many will consider that questions about cardiotocographs are unfair in a DRCOG examination. Visually they make good OSCE stations so do not be surprised if you see them. The five traces shown are classic.

In validation, approximately 30% of candidates described the correct physiological mechanism. Only 2% picked the correct trace!

B➤ 1. Trace B (baseline tachycardia alone with no other features) — **1**

2. a Midstream urine/catheter sample for microscopy and culture — **1**
   b Maternal blood cultures — **1**
   c High vaginal swab or 'clean catch' of liquor for microscopy and culture — **1**

Most candidates have managed to pick the correct trace. The tests requested are obviously those that would be performed to investigate a maternal pyrexia.

Howlers! Ultrasound; blood pressure recordings; urea and electrolytes.

C➤ 1. Trace E (tachycardia, loss of baseline variability, persistent late decelerations) — **1**

2. Significant foetal hypoxia — **1**
3. Foetal blood sampling — **1**

Most candidates have picked the correct trace. When stating what it represents, foetal distress is not acceptable as all traces show this to some degree.

D➤ Cord compression — **1**

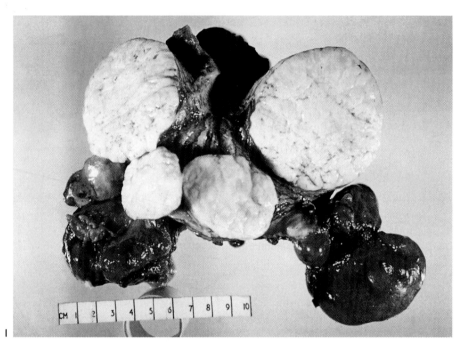

I

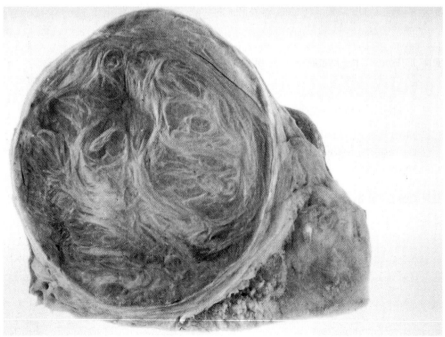

II

QUESTIONS

Score

A➤ Study photograph I.

  1. What condition does it show?

  _____

  2. List two characteristic appearances of this condition.

  a _____

  b _____

B➤ 1. What percentage of this condition undergoes sarcomatous change?

  _____ %

  2. How do sarcomatous changes present?

  _____

C➤ 1. What complication is depicted in photograph II.

  _____

  2. Explain the patho-aetiology.

  _____

  3. How does this present clinically?

  _____

  4. List two other conditions that one should consider as a differential diagnosis in a woman presenting with this condition.

  1. _____

  2. _____

ANSWERS/COMMENTS

	Score

A➤ 1. Multiple fibroids   **1**

2. Any two of the following: **2**
   a White, raised cut surface
   b Classic whorled cut surface
   c Well circumscribed – there is a false capsule of compressed uterine muscle (allows easy enucleation at surgery)

1. In validation, two thirds of candidates have identified the condition correctly as fibroids.

 Howlers! Polycystic ovaries; carcinoma of the cervix; vaginal carcinoma.

2. *Differentiator: Despite a good quality photograph, only 15% of candidates have been able to give two macroscopic appearances of a fibroid.*

B➤ 1. Less than 1%   **1**

2. Abdominal pain, rapid growth   **1**

A wide range of answers have been suggested. We suspect most candidates just had a guess.

Leiomyosarcomas are rare tumours. Malignant degeneration of a fibroid accounts for half of them, but they may arise from normal myometrium or endometrial stroma. Most patients are between 40 and 60 years of age. The commonst symptoms are abnormal vaginal bleeding and abdominal pain. Treatment is surgical. Radiotherapy is relatively ineffective. The five-year survival rate is approximately 45% for stage I disease, falling to 30% for stage II.

ANSWERS/COMMENTS

	Score

C➤ 1. Necrobiosis (red degeneration) — **1**

2. Occurs typically during pregnancy. Rapid growth of the fibroid (secondary to raised endogenous oestrogen levels) leads to infarction of the centre of the tumour. — **1**

3. Sudden enlargement of the fibroid, which becomes tender and painful — **1**

4. Any two of the following: — **2**
   - a Placental abruption
   - b On the right – acute appendicitis
   - c Torsion of an ovarian cyst

Less than 10% of candidates have recognized this as red degeneration.

A photograph of a normal fibroid in cross-section is present for comparison. The normal fibroid looks white.

QUESTIONS

Initial flow rate   18 ml/s
Volume voided   230 ml
Residual   30 ml

Early 1st desire to void at 180 ml
Urgency reported at 350 ml
Maximum cystometric capacity was 490 ml

Stable bladder; with normal compliance
Detrusor pressure at end of filling: 11 cmH_2O

Bladder outline normal, with no reflux
Bladder base low at rest, with further descent on coughing
Marked incontinence seen

Voiding pressure mounted was 25 cmH_2O
Difficulty in 'stopping mid-stream', voided with flow rates of 23 ml/s and residual of 50 ml

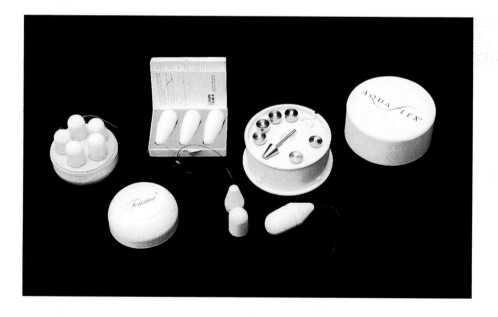

QUESTIONS

Study Mrs Forbes-Smythe's videocystography report (she is aged 42 years).

A➤ What is the diagnosis in this case?

_____

B➤ If a conservative approach to management is adopted:

1. What would be the *improvement* rate?

_____

2. How long would it take to see an improvement?

_____

C➤ Study the object in front of you.

1. What is it?

_____

2. What advantage does it offer?

_____

D➤ What surgical treatment options are available?

1. _____

2. _____

E➤ What is a pad test?

_____

ANSWERS/COMMENTS

	Score

A➤ Genuine stress incontinence   **2**

In validation, most candidates gave the correct answer. One candidate offered a diagnosis of cystocoele – hard to achieve with no examination findings!

B➤ 1. 50–70%   **1**
2. 4–6 months   **1**

In validation, over half the candidates answered incorrectly. Most badly underestimated how long it would take to achieve an improvement in the problem.

C➤ 1. Vaginal cone   **1**

 Howlers! Transducer; rectal pressure gauge; intrauterine contraceptive.

2. Increases patient compliance rate/biofeedback   **1**

This has been poorly answered. Answers such as 'conservative approach' or 'avoids surgery' will not be accepted. Any physiotherapy will achieve this. Need to be specific to the advantage of cones.

 Howler! Comfortable fit.

ANSWERS/COMMENTS

Score
2

D► Any two of the following:

1. Vaginal anterior repair
2. Colposuspension ·
3. Stamey/Raz/Perera
4. Vesica bladder stabilization procedure
5. Periurethral collagen injections
6. Transvaginal tape (TVT)

Vaginal hysterectomy without a repair is not an acceptable answer because it is the repair that is needed to achieve continence.

A few gynaecologists would prefer a sling as primary procedure but this is not standard.

We have included as complete a list of surgical options as possible. The colposuspension is still the 'gold standard', offering a 90–95% dry rate at the end of year 1. The anterior repair is not nearly as successful or long lasting (75% dry at the end of year 1, dropping to less than 50% at five years). The needles procedures (Stamey, Raz, Perera) have been largely discredited in recent studies – some quoting only 20% dry rate at year 5). The Vesica, laparoscopic colposuspension and periurethral injections are newer techniques. Long-term data are not yet available. Nevertheless, you were only asked to give surgical treatment options – not to justify or grade them.

E► Allows you to quantify the urinary loss. Pads are worn for 24 hours and weighed (both dry and wet) to allow calculation.

2

Most candidates have said 'if the pad is wet'. You must include in your answer reference to weighing the pad or quantifying urinary loss.

 Tip: Questions A and E are examples of weighted answers. Question A deserves more marks because it requires the candidate to interpret data. Question E requires a full definition. Only one mark is given if only half the information is provided.

REST STATION

QUESTIONS

Score

You are approached by your community midwife who is keen to establish parentcraft classes in your practice. She asks you to join her.

A➤ List four key topics which should be covered by these classes specifically related to labour.

1. _____

2. _____

3. _____

4. _____

B➤ List four topics related to the postnatal period that should be discussed.

1. _____

2. _____

3. _____

4. _____

C➤ At the first parentcraft class, a patient says her husband has epilepsy. You are asked if this is a contraindication to vaccinating this child with pertussis.

Yes/No _____

D➤ Another mother asks you on what day the midwife usually finishes visiting at home after delivery.

_____

ANSWERS/COMMENTS

Score

A► 1. Signs of onset of labour | 1

and any three of the following: | 3

2. Pain relief
3. Relaxation
4. Labour and delivery positions
5. Tour of delivery suite

Signs of onset of labour is a vital piece of information that must be communicated to all parents-to-be. Most candidates have included types of analgesia, relaxation and breathing exercises and delivery positions. The tour of the labour ward is also important so that surroundings are familiar to the patient on arrival.

B► 1. Feeding | 1

and any three of the following: | 3

2. Handling/bathing the baby
3. Immunizations
4. Pelvic floor exercises
5. Care of the perineum

Discussion regarding infant feeding is probably the most important area to cover. Immunization is also an important topic.

The signs of onset of labour and infant feeding are required as essential answers. A mark is lost if they are not included. This is an example of a compulsory answer. Currently, the RCOG does not include this form in the examination but it is included here to illustrate other possible marking schemes.

C► No | 1

Most candidates have suggested the correct answer.

D► Day 10 | 1

Surprisingly, several candidates have offered six weeks as the answer.

INTERACTIVE STATION

Score

Instructions to candidate

Rose Hughes, aged 44 years, has attended your surgery for consultation. She is new to the area and you have not seen her before.

She has a number of complaints that she will outline in detail.

Conduct the interview as you would in your surgery, answering her questions as appropriate.

By the end of the interview she should feel confident that you have understood the nature of her problem and have a management plan.

Instructions to actress

You are a 44-year-old lady suffering from severe PMT. During the interview with the candidate you must appear agitated and tense. At times you are almost aggressive, demanding attention and frequently gripping the doctor's arm.

You have a long list of continual complaints: you can't cope at work/you hate your husband, he just does not understand you/the kids are getting on top of you/you are taken for granted, no-one ever helps around the house/you have terrible breast tenderness before periods/you feel bloated all the time, etc.

Somewhere in this diatribe you must include the following important facts: you were unable to take the pill for contraception due to bad headaches/you do feel well for just ten days a month, after your period/ you feel so 'low' sometimes you have considered leaving home, just walking out/you attacked your husband with a carving knife three months ago, when you were really uptight.

You want to know:
What is the problem?
The reasons for the doctor's diagnosis of the problem.
What test can be done?
What treatments can be offered?
Which treatment is best for me?

ANSWERS/COMMENTS

	Score

Marks allocated by the actress

Appropriate eye contact	1
Listened attentively	1
Confidence in candidate	1
I would like to see this person again	1

Marks allocated by the examiner

Correct diagnosis made	1
Correct reasons given	1
Correct tests outlined	1
Treatment options discussed	1
Sensible approach for this individual patient	1
Difficult interview handled well	1

Facts to include

Diagnosis PMT

Cyclical nature of symptoms – clear 'window' when asymptomatic, lasting at least one week

PMT chart – patient to keep monthly calendar of symptoms. These should be cyclical.

Mainly a diagnosis by exclusion

Thyroid function tests

Follicle-stimulating hormone should be performed.

(Florid PMT can be confused with perimenopause in mid-40s.)

Treatment options include

Dietary approach

Non-hormonal approach, pyridoxine and oil of evening primrose

Low-dose contraceptive pill

Hormone replacement therapy – high-dose patches or implants

Cyclical progestogens – Provera/Duphaston

Cyclical progesterone, i.e. Cyclogest

Fluoxatine

GnRh analogues

Clinical psychologist/stress management strategies

ANSWERS/COMMENTS

It would be best to start with a non-hormonal approach using high doses of pyridoxine hydrochloride (vitamin B_6) and oil of evening primrose (200 mg a day and 1000–1500 mg a day respectively). Because the patient is unstable it would be acceptable to give high doses of vitamin B_6 for a short time, reducing the dose to a 50 mg maintenance level. Studies have shown that prolonged high doses of B_6 can cause reversible nerve toxicity in rats. The patient has symptoms of progestogen sensitivity, for example mastalgia and bloating. She also suffered from bad headaches whilst taking the combined pill. Therefore, it is best to avoid hormonal treatment, at least in the first instance. In view of her aggression, fluoxatine may be helpful here. If hormonal treatment became necessary it would be preferable to commence hormone replacement therapy, thus utilizing natural rather than synthetic oestrogens.

Although this was a very straightforward station, the performance range was still very variable. Range of marks 4–10, mean 8.2, standard deviation 1.8.

Most candidates arrived at the correct diagnosis and commented on the cyclical nature of symptoms. Fewer candidates suggested the use of a PMT chart to monitor the pattern of symptoms. Those candidates who did badly made little attempt to describe the treatment options available and did not have a logical approach to the management of this particular patient.

QUESTIONS

Philippa Stebbings is 28 years of age and a clinical psychologist. She makes an appointment to see you, having performed two pregnancy tests which are both positive. This is her first pregnancy and she and her husband Donald are delighted. You calculate she is six weeks pregnant.

A➤ List four general topics you would aim to cover in this consultation.

1.

2.

3.

4.

B➤ Philippa informs you that two years ago she suffered her first episode of genital herpes. She understands this could potentially be a problem. She has experienced three recurrent attacks in the last 18 months. What advice would you give her regarding:

1. need for antenatal screening tests?

2. mode of delivery?

3. risk associated with epidural analgesia in labour?

QUESTIONS

C➤ Donald's cousin recently had a baby diagnosed as having Tay–Sachs. Philippa and Donald are Jews.

1. What is the underlying deficiency in Tay–Sachs disease?

2. What advice would you give about identifying the baby's risk?

3. What is the mode of inheritance?

ANSWERS/COMMENTS

	Score

A➤ Any four of the following: **4**

1. Exploring her anxieties
2. Discuss folate supplements
3. Where she would like to have the baby
4. Full medical history to identify any risk factor
5. Arrange for her booking bloods to be taken
6. General advice re early pregnancy
7. Discuss diet (including salmonella/listeria)
8. Provide written information about pregnancy
9. Discuss maternity leave if relevant

This is a very broad question and therefore there are many acceptable answers. You should pick up maximum marks here! This is an important visit. The couple are normally full of optimism and excitement. How this consultation is handled will set the scene for the whole of the pregnancy. It will uncover any potential areas for concern and help to ensure the most appropriate care is given.

B➤ 1. Nothing to worry about – no tests needed   **1**
    2. Vaginal delivery unless active lesions at time of delivery   **1**
    3. Minimal risk of herpetic encephalitis (risk often overrated)   **1**

During validation, this section was surprisingly well answered.

Herpes simplex virus (HSV) type 2 causes 70% of herpetic genital tract infections. Diagnosis is by culture in a special viral culture medium or by electron microscopy of vesicular scrapings. Acyclovir has proved very useful in reducing discomfort from vulval lesions in the non-pregnant case and can be used in pregnancy as well.

In the past vaginal swabs were perfomed weekly from 36 weeks' gestation until delivery. This is now no longer performed. There is no risk to the foetus unless active lesions are present at the time of delivery.

The foetus has no intrinsic immunity to HSV. Although vaginal delivery in the presence of active lesions may not lead to foetal infection, 50% of affected infants die. Therefore, the policy would still be to perform a caesarean section in these circumstances, as long as the membranes remain intact or have been ruptured less than four hours ago. There have been some documented cases of foetal infection even when caesarean sections have been performed. Primary lesions are the most infective and, of course, occur without warning, so are the most dangerous. Recurrent attacks are much less infective and the sufferer usually knows what to expect so action can be taken.

ANSWERS/COMMENTS

	Score
C▶ 1. Glucosidase deficiency (a deficiency of β-hexosaminidase, more precisely)	**1**
2. Parents can both be screened initially for carrier status	**1**
3. Autosomal recessive	**1**

Part 1 requires a specific answer; 'enzyme deficiency' is not sufficient.

Many candidates have answered 'chorionic villus sampling' for part 2. Tay–Sachs is an autosomal recessive disorder so both parents can be screened to check carrier status. This avoids the need to perform an invasive test on the foetus which has a significant risk of miscarriage.

Two disorders, Lesch–Nyhan syndrome and Tay–Sachs disease, have been investigated extensively with a view to the use of enzyme microassays for preimplantation diagnosis in the human. Initial experimentation in mice looked promising but in humans this technique looks unlikely to be useful for preimplantation diagnosis of inherited enzyme deficiencies.

QUESTIONS

Score

Mrs Smithers attends for her routine antenatal check at 24 weeks. During the consultation she asks about maternity benefits. She is clearly unsure of her entitlement.

A▶ 1. How many weeks before the expected time of delivery can 'maternity leave' be said to begin?

_____ weeks

2. For how many weeks is pay usually maintained at the full rate?

_____ weeks

3. For how many weeks is pay reduced to half rate?

_____ weeks

B▶ 1. What form needs to be completed before maternity pay can be started?

_____

2. Who can complete this form?

_____

3. What information (apart from patient details) is required on the form?

_____

C▶ List two potential physical work hazards in pregnancy.

1. _____

2. _____

D▶ List two potential chemical hazards to pregnancy found at work.

1. _____

2. _____

ANSWERS/COMMENTS

	Score
A► 1. 11 weeks	1
2. 6 weeks	1
3. 12 weeks	1

> **D** **Differentiator:** *In validation, this question was very poorly answered with less than 10% of candidates giving the correct answer. This is basic information that a general practitioner should know.*

	Score
B► 1. MAT.B1	1
2. Doctor or midwife	1
3. Expected date of confinement	1

Usually this section has been answered well.

C►ꞏ Any two of the following: **2**

1. Noise
2. Vibration
3. Heat
4. Humidity
5. Repetitive VDU work
6. Lifting heavy loads
7. Dust
8. Ionizing radiation, e.g. X-rays

Candidates have offered antepartum haemorrhage and preterm labour. You are specifically asked for physical work hazards in pregnancy – these are complications, not physical hazards.

D►ꞏ Any two of the following: **2**

1. Metals, e.g. lead, mercury, copper
2. Gases, e.g. carbon monoxide
3. Passive smoking
4. Herbicides, solvents, e.g. carbon tetrachloride
5. Drugs during manufacturing
6. Disinfecting agents, e.g. ethylene oxide

This question has been very poorly answered.

> **Tip:** *Many gave X-rays but this is not a chemical hazard. You must read the question carefully.*

QUESTIONS

Umbilical cord prolapse is an obstetric emergency.

A➤ What is the pathophysiology of foetal distress following a cord prolapse?

B➤ List three clinical conditions that predispose to cord prolapse.

1.

2.

3.

C➤ The emergency management of a cord prolapse may include:

1. elevation of the presenting part out of the pelvis.

   Yes/No

2. placing the mother in the knee–chest position.

   Yes/No

3. filling the bladder with 700 ml of saline.

   Yes/No

4. placing the mother in the left lateral position.

   Yes/No

5. placing the mother in the Trendelenberg position.

   Yes/No

6. wrapping the cord in a warm swab.

   Yes/No

ANSWERS/COMMENTS

	Score

A➤ 1. Vasospasm due to cooling

or

2. Compression to the cord

1

Compression of the cord has been the answer most commonly given. Some candidates offered 'hypoxia'. This is too non-specific.

Vasospasm due to cooling of the exposed cord is probably the most important factor in causing foetal distress. This was seldom given as the answer.

B➤ Any three of the following:

3

1. Breech presentation
2. Twin pregnancy
3. Prematurity
4. Grand multiparity
5. Transverse lie
6. Placenta praevia (not covering the cervical os)
7. Polyhydramnios

 Pitfall: *Malpresentation is too vague. An occipitoposterior presentation or a brow presentation fits well into the pelvis and hence is not associated with cord prolapse.*

 Howler! *Shoulder dystocia.*

C➤ 1. Yes **1**
2. Yes **1**
3. Yes **1**
4. No **1**
5. Yes **1**
6. Yes **1**

Parts 1, 2, 3 and 5 will all help to elevate the presenting part and reduce cord compression. Keeping the cord warm will reduce the risk of vasospasm.

QUESTIONS

A 29-year-old Australian mother attends your antenatal clinic at 34 weeks' gestation. She had an ultrasound two days before because the placenta was low lying at her 20-week anomaly scan. The placenta is no longer covering the cervix.

She asks you to look at the growth chart which is in her notes as she is not due to be reviewed at the hospital antenatal clinic for another two weeks. The growth chart is attached.

A➤ What does this show?

_____

_____

B➤ List four possible groups of causes of these ultrasound findings.

1. _____

2. _____

3. _____

4. _____

C➤ List two further ultrasound features that might differentiate between these causes.

1. _____

2. _____

D➤ 1. What is the most appropriate antenatal screening procedure in this case?

_____

_____

2. What two specific tests in this screening procedure will enable a positive diagnosis to be made?

a _____

b _____

QUESTIONS

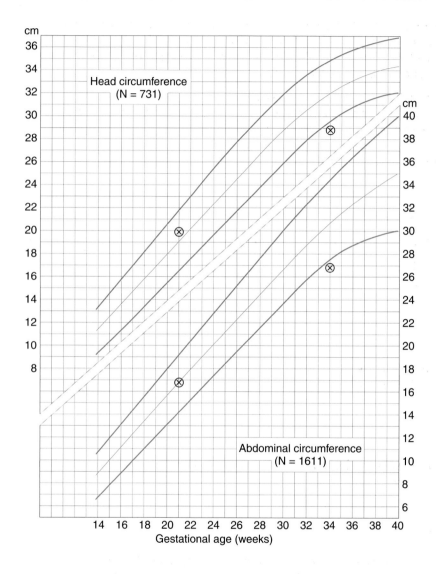

ANSWERS/COMMENTS

Score

A▶ Symmetrical growth retardation

1

This question aroused much anger from some candidates who commented that general practitioners are not asked to comment on ultrasound growth charts in a primary care setting. Nevertheless, we felt this to be a fair question. Virtually all general practitioners have performed six months of obstetrics and gynaecology at some time as part of their training, and must have some basic idea as to the difference between symmetrical and asymmetrical growth retardation since the aetiology is very different and certainly affects management. All general practitioners, whether they decide to be GP obstetricians and take on home deliveries or not, will be doing a lot more antenatal care in the future. For this reason we have left the question intact.

Differentiator: *Only 50–60% of candidates have answered this correctly. The rest have been rather vague, offering an answer of 'growth retardation'. We felt that this was not specific enough. The whole point of the question was to test the candidate's ability to recognize the two different types of growth retardation. Pregnancy-induced hypertension causes asymmetical growth retardation. There is head sparing for as long as possible and only in situations of extreme malnourishment do the biparietal diameter and head circumference begin to fall off.*

B▶ Any four of the following:

4

1. Chromosomal anomalies
2. Transplacental viral infections, e.g. rubella, toxoplasma
3. Smoking
4. Alcohol
5. Certain drugs

The majority of candidates completed two out of four parts correctly. Approximately 11% got three out of four parts correct. Some candidates have offered 'infection' as one of the possible causes for symmetrical growth retardation. We felt this was not specific enough. Obviously, it is transplacental viral infection that is the cause. Several candidates have offered three different types of transplacental viral infections, e.g. rubella, toxoplasmosis, cytomegalovirus, rather than offering different types of causation for symmetrical growth retardation. It is extremely hard when writing OSCE questions to iron out absolutely all ambiguity in the stem but we felt that the stem was in fact as specific as we could make it and therefore, after deliberation,

ANSWERS/COMMENTS

Score

we decided against accepting lists of viral infections as this was really demonstrating that the candidate could not think of any other causes to account for the problem.

 Pitfall: *Although wrong dates might account for the appearance on the growth chart, in real life it is rather stupid to offer this as an answer during an examination. This is an example of being too clever and coming to grief because of it. If you are given a stem containing information then you must assume that the information is accurate and correct.*

C► 1. Ultrasound markers of infection, i.e. cerebral calcification   1
2. Ultrasound markers for major congenital anomalies, i.e. septal   1
 defects, hepatosplenomegaly, low-set ears

A lot of candidates gave very generalized answers that had nothing to do with the question posed. Liquor volume estimation, estimated birth weight and Doppler blood flow studies are all different examples of tests to see, either directly, or indirectly, if there is poor placental perfusion and placental insufficiency. The question had asked for specific features that might distinguish between the causes of symmetrical growth retardation, i.e. chromosomal causes and viral infections, so that these answers were way off the theme.

D► 1. Cordocentesis   1
2. a Chromosomal analysis   1
 b Serum IgM assay   1

Surprisingly few candidates had any idea about cordocentesis. When we initially piloted the question we asked what was the most appropriate antenatal screening investigation. This was deemed to be too difficult and the validation process showed the candidates really had not considered cordocentesis as an answer at all. Therefore this particular stem was changed. Nevertheless, the level of knowledge of cordocentesis as a procedure for in vivo foetal sampling has been poor.

QUESTIONS

Hysterectomy is a very commonly performed operation. It is associated with well-recognized short-term and long-term complications.

A▶ Which procedure is associated with lower morbidity, total abdominal hysterectomy or vaginal hysterectomy?

B▶ List three measures that are currently in routine practice to reduce the incidence of postoperative deep venous thrombosis for all hysterectomies.

1.

2.

3.

C▶ What other general important prophylactic measure should be taken in all cases of hysterectomy?

D▶ Should the patient be given an enema preoperatively before a routine hysterectomy?

Yes/No

E▶ In a fit 47-year-old, what preoperative investigations would you order?

1.

2.

F▶ When would you expect vaginal bleeding to finish following routine hysterectomy?

G▶ When can a woman return to work following a routine vaginal hysterectomy?

ANSWERS/COMMENTS

	Score
A► **Vaginal**	1

B► **Any three of the following:** 3

1. TED stockings
2. Flotrons
3. Subcutaneous anticoagulant
4. Early mobilization

While it is correct to stop the combined oral contraceptive pill before surgery, this answer is not acceptable in the context of this question. The stem specifically asks for measures that are currently routine practice, used in all cases. Stopping the pill is only relevant to the patient currently taking it.

C► **Antibiotics at the time of induction** 1

The majority of candidates have answered this as if the stem referred back to question B, attempting to give further measures to reduce the incidence of deep venous thrombosis. We have already asked for three measures to reduce the incidence of deep venous thrombosis. This should alert candidates to the fact that this question was asking for a different facet of prophylaxis.

Tip: The same answer is not needed twice.

Many candidates introduced important issues such as better surgical technique and shorter anaesthetic time, but these are not 'prophylactic measures'.

D► **No** 1

E► **Any two of the following:** 2

1. Full blood count
2. Blood group
3. Request that serum sample is saved

Pitfall: 'Fit' is the key word in this question, therefore investigations such as clotting screen, scans, ultrasound will not be accepted.

ANSWERS/COMMENTS

Score

F➤ 3–6 weeks   **1**

In validation, virtually all candidates gave the wrong answer; 70% said that the bleeding stopped after a week or less. Although bleeding is often light and intermittent it can continue for up to six weeks. Frequently, it increases as the vaginal stitches begin to dissolve, 2–4 weeks after surgery.

G➤ 4–6 weeks   **1**

This question has been poorly answered.

 Tip: Questions F and G test basic gynaecological knowledge which GPs must know to counsel their patients accurately.

QUESTIONS

Mrs Jones has just delivered a 4600 g boy, her fifth child, at home. The attending midwife gave intramuscular syntometrine but Mrs Jones still sustained a postpartum haemorrhage of 1500 ml. She is not yet clinically shocked. The senior midwife has sited a Venflon and taken bloods for crossmatch.

A➤ List four key stages you would undertake to manage Mrs Jones.

1.

2.

3.

4.

B➤ Define primary postpartum haemorrhage.

C➤ In general obstetric practice list the four main causes of primary postpartum haemorrhage.

1.

2.

3.

4.

ANSWERS/COMMENTS

	Score
A➤ 1. Rub up a uterine contraction.	1
2. Give ergometrine.	1
3. Start an intravenous infusion of Hartmann's.	1
4. Determine the cause and deal with it appropriately.	1

This question has been very poorly answered, but it is a fair question. With the Cumberlege recommendations, Mrs Jones might well be delivering at home since she is a multiparous patient. Some knowledge of initial emergency procedures is necessary. You are told that a venflon has been sited but not that an infusion was started. Many candidates did not give this answer. Read the question! Haemobate or Pg F2α would only be given in a hospital setting and were not accepted.

 Howler! Consent for laparotomy and hysterectomy.

B➤ Loss of 500 ml or more of blood within 24 hours of delivery   **2**
(1 mark for volume lost; 1 mark for the time interval)

Surprisingly, less than 50% of candidates have given the correct answer to this question. Volumes varied from 1000 ml to as little as 250 ml; others did not quantify blood loss at all. Many did not stipulate the time interval after delivery.

C➤ 1. Retained placenta	1
2. Uterine atony	1
3. Genital tract tears	1
4. Coagulation defect	1

Generally this question has been answered well and most candidates gave three out of four correct answers.

Some candidates listed cervical tears and vaginal tears as separate answers. These are all included under the heading of genital tract tears. By asking for 'four main causes', it was intended that the different factors which may contribute to postpartum haemorrhage should be listed.

 Howler! Antepartum haemorrhage.

QUESTIONS

You are called to see a baby who has just been delivered at 32 weeks' gestation following a rapid labour.

A► List four signs of respiratory distress in the newborn.

1.

2.

3.

4.

B► What antenatal treatment can be used to reduce the risk of respiratory disease (doses must be included)?

C► List four non-pulmonary causes of respiratory distress that need to be considered in a baby delivered at 36 weeks with respiratory distress.

1.

2.

3.

4.

D► Prematurity accounts for only 10% of births. What percentage of first-week neonatal deaths can be attributed to this?

%

ANSWERS/COMMENTS

Score

A➤ Any four of the following: 4

1. Tachypnoea 60 breaths/min
2. Expiratory grunting
3. Subcostal, intercostal recession
4. Cyanosis
5. Alar flaring

This question has been well answered. Most candidates had three out of four correct. Twenty percent of candidates mentioned the accessory muscles but only adults can 'fix' their pectoral girdle.

B➤ 12 mg betamethasone or dexamethasone, given in two doses, 12–24 hours apart   1

Disturbingly, 70% of candidates just gave the answer 'steroids'. This is not specific enough when the question asked for the dose to be given.

 Tip: It is important to read the question carefully.

C➤ Any four of the following: 4

1. Congenital heart disease
2. Acute anaemia
3. Polycythaemia
4. Metabolic acidosis
5. Birth trauma including intraventricular haemorrhage
6. Septicaemia
7. Diaphragmatic hernia

Since only four non-pulmonary causes of distress were requested, this was a generous question. One candidate suggested 'incorrect dates', presumably indicating respiratory distress syndrome secondary to prematurity. If the stem quotes 36 weeks as being the gestation, it is sensible to believe it. Diabetes would precipitate upper respiratory tract infections or respiratory distress syndrome, i.e. it would precipitate *pulmonary* causes. Meconium aspiration is also a *pulmonary* cause.

D➤ 60–70%   1

This question has not been answered as well as expected. Several candidates suggested only 20–30%.

 Howler! One candidate thought that prematurity accounted for only 1% of neonatal deaths!

REST STATION

INTERACTIVE STATION

Instructions to candidate

You have known Nora Black for some years and have always found her to be rather demanding and difficult. She was not at all happy with the outcome of her first pregnancy, a forceps delivery, at 39 weeks and four days' gestation.

Nora, aged 37 years, is now 38 weeks into her second pregnancy and fully expects a home confinement. Your midwife has warned you that she thinks this is a breech presentation.

Your examination today confirms a breech presentation and you feel that the baby may be bigger than the last one (birth weight 7 lb 5 oz). You are *not* happy to manage this baby at home.

Please conduct the interview accordingly, answering Mrs Black's questions and explaining in full your concerns.

Instructions to actress

You are Nora Black, a rather big-boned, 37-year-old shop assistant who has always had a domineering personality.

Your first child was delivered by lift-out forceps at 39 weeks and four days' gestation, weighing 7 lb 5 oz. You maintain that the hospital interfered too soon and that you would have had a normal vaginal delivery if you had been left to push longer. You still harbour a suspicion that the junior registrar involved needed forceps practice!

You have therefore insisted on a home confinement this time and have visited the hospital as little as possible, being seen mainly by your GP and the community midwife.

You are now at 38 weeks' gestation and the midwife has asked you to see the doctor because she is sure this is a breech presentation. The following discussion takes place after the doctor has confirmed this finding.

You need to adopt a very abrasive and dominant approach. You need to make it clear you have *not* changed your mind and that you do not expect the findings to make any difference. You will repeatedly remind the doctor of the last delivery outcome. You will enquire about the problems of breech delivery, about the risks of home delivery in this case, if any tests can be done to prove home confinement would be safe, and finally if there are any compromise arrangements that can be made.

INTERACTIVE STATION

If the candidate conducts the interview well, you will be prepared to listen to reason and compromise in the end.

Instructions to examiner

This station tests the candidate's ability to handle a difficult and somewhat aggressive patient in a professional and courteous manner, whilst clearly stating his/her professional concerns regarding the proposed mode of delivery. A clear succinct argument should be offered together with a well-developed alternative plan of management. A candidate who allows the actress to 'browbeat' him/her into submission or who demonstrates irritability has done badly.

ANSWERS/COMMENTS

	Score

Marks awarded by the actress

Appropriate eye contact	1
Listened attentively	1
Confidence in candidate	1
I would like to see this person again	1

Marks awarded by the examiner

Non-confrontational (did not alienate patient)	1
Good listening skills (acknowledged patient's anger and frustration)	1
Good explanations of risks of breech delivery given	1
Risks of home delivery adequately explained	1
Suitable alternative management explained, e.g. DOMINO delivery	1
Maintained professional stance (did not allow patient to alter candidate's professional opinion)	1

This interactive station demonstrated the technique of altering the conversation based on the candidate's performance. In certain situations the outcome of the conversation will depend on how the actress responds to the candidate. Actresses will be instructed to continue to be difficult, argumentative patients or to become more co-operative and compliant depending on whether they feel the candidate is performing well and has some grasp of the subject under discussion. Range of marks 2–10, mean 8, standard deviation 1.9.

There has been a very wide range of response to this station and some candidates performed very badly. Usually, this was either because the candidate took a confrontational stance and alienated the patient who then, of course, became as unco-operative as possible or because he/she was unable to stand his/her ground and justify his/her position in refusing a home delivery in this case.

Several candidates have been unable to offer an alternative management plan or explain the risks of home delivery adequately.

QUESTIONS

Score

A 50-year-old patient attends your surgery in a state of panic. Her sister, aged 47 years, has just been diagnosed and treated for ovarian carcinoma and is now undertaking chemotherapy following her hysterectomy and bilateral oophorectomy.

A➤ She would like to know if her chances of ovarian cancer are higher than average.

Yes/No

B➤ She last had a smear one year ago, which was normal. She now demands another. Would you recommend one?

Yes/No

C➤ What two general screening tests are available for ovarian cancers?

1. _____

2. _____

D➤ At the end of her consultation, the patient confides in a whisper that her mother also died of ovarian cancer at the age of 56 years. Will her estimated increased risk of developing ovarian cancer above the general population be:

1. 15%?

    Yes/No

2. 20%?

    Yes/No

3. 35%?

    Yes/No

4. 50%

    Yes/No

E➤ Would there be an increased risk of the disease if the *only* family member to have had ovarian cancer was a cousin?

Yes/No

QUESTIONS

F➤ The patient begs you to refer her for hysterectomy and removal of both her ovaries. Do you consider that her family history (mother and sister) is an indication for surgery?

Yes/No

ANSWERS/COMMENTS

	Score
A▶ Yes	1
B▶ No	1

We have been surprised at how well this station has been answered, with 100% of candidates giving correct answers for A and 90% correct for B. Obviously, cervical smears only screen for cervical dysplasia and squamous carcinoma. There is no relation or relevance to ovarian carcinoma.

C▶ 1. Pelvic ultrasound (preferably using a vaginal probe)   1
    2. Tumour marks, e.g. CA125 α-fetoprotein   1

All candidates have suggested ultrasound and have gained one mark. The use of a vaginal probe increases the sensitivity of this test. We could have insisted that the vaginal probe was included in the answer to make it more difficult. The examination board at the college can decide to alter the marking scheme for a station in a future examination if they feel the original one was too easy. Usually the question is withdrawn and repiloted first.

If candidates answered 'tumour markers' or gave a specific example of a tumour marker, a mark was awarded. However, candidates who gave examples of two tumour markers but failed to give ultrasound scored only one mark.

Pitfall: *A small number of candidates have answered 'gene probes'. These can be used to look for Lynch type II families which are linked to ovarian carcinoma. However, this technique would not be used to screen the general population.*

D▶ 1. No   1
    2. No   1
    3. Yes   1
    4. No   1

Differentiator: *Only 35% of candidates have offered the correct answer. Most have felt that the risk was 50%.*

E▶ No	1
F▶ Yes	1

These questions have been answered well with 85% and 95% correct answers respectively.

QUESTIONS

A 15-year-old girl is brought to your surgery by her very anxious mother. Christina has not yet started menstruating and is wondering why she is different from other girls at school. She is not sexually active.

A► Outline two relevant questions you would need to include in your history taking.

1. _____

2. _____

B► List four relevant features you would look for or exclude during your physical examination.

1. _____

2. _____

3. _____

4. _____

C► List two tests that you would organize.

1. _____

2. _____

D► What is the most likely diagnosis?

_____

E► What treatment would you offer?

_____

ANSWERS/COMMENTS

Score
2

A➤ Any two of the following:

1. At what age did your mother and/or sisters have their menarche?
2. Is Christina exhibiting any monthly cyclical pains?
3. Has Christina had any marked weight loss (dietary fads/anorexia)?
4. Ask about other signs of puberty.

All candidates did well. Most mentioned sudden weight loss and family history of delayed puberty. Several asked if there were other signs of delayed puberty. Cyclical pain was mentioned by only one candidate.

The possibility of stress at home or school was mentioned once. This is more likely to result in missed periods rather than totally delayed puberty.

B➤ Any four of the following:

4

1. Height/weight
2. Breast development and body hair distribution
3. Nipple spacing
4. Wide carrying angle
5. Normal genitalia – clitoromegaly
6. Intact hymen, but patent vaginal opening
7. Hirsutism

Obviously this stem is designed to test the candidate's ability to think of differential diagnoses and ask the pertinent questions necessary to distinguish between them.

- Looking at the body mass index (height and weight) demarcates the anorexic.
- Adrenogenital syndrome is excluded by inspection of the external genitalia.
- Sex organ unresponsiveness (i.e. genetically male child with undescended testes and poor sensitivity to testoterone might be considered with no breast development and ambiguous genitalia.
- Turner syndrome often present with short stature, wide nipple spacing and wide carrying angle.
- Haematocolpos will demonstrate a blue bulge, with blood products building up behind an intact hymen.

Most candidates got at least three out of four. Two candidates offered visual field defects and one mentioned nipple discharge, obviously considering a prolactinoma. This would be very unlikely in a 15 year old with primary amenorrhoea.

ANSWERS/COMMENTS

Some candidates offered breast development, axillary hair distribution and pubic hair distribution as three separate answers. These answers all cover one differential, and have not demonstrated an ability to think of other causes of this condition or to try to exclude/prove them.

Tip: Try to think why the question has been asked and what the examiners want to test.

C➤ 1. Pelvic ultrasound

    2. LH, FSH

1

1

Most candidates listed the correct tests.

D➤ Normal variation.

1

The next most likely cause is polycystic ovarian syndrome, which affects approximately 15% of teenagers.

E➤ No treatment. Reassurance is all that is necessary.

1

Most candidates agreed that Christina's amenorrhoea represented a normal variation and were not proactive at this stage. She should be advised to keep her weight steady, eat a healthy diet and exercise. The body mass index (BMI) is relevant. She should be reviewed in one year's time and if she has not started menstruating, a progestogen challenge test should be implemented.

QUESTIONS

A▶ For legal purposes what are the four notifiable diseases that suggest recent sexual encounters?

1. _____

2. _____

3. _____

4. _____

B▶ 1. The normal treatment for gonorrhoea is an IM injection of 4/8 megaunits of procaine penicillin.

True/False

2. The prevalence of penicillin-resistant strains of gonorrhoea is 4% in London.

True/False

3. The incidence of syphilis has remained static for the last five years.

True/False

4. *Neisseria gonorrhoeae* is isolated from a high vaginal swab.

True/False

C▶ What other aspect of treatment of sexually transmitted disease is vitally important?

_____

D▶ What do you understand by the term 'Double Dutch'?

_____

ANSWERS/COMMENTS

	Score
A► 1. Gonorrhoea	1
2. Aphilitic chancre or primary syphilis	1
3. Chancroid	1
4. Lymphogranuloma venereum (LGV)	1

This was poorly attempted with no candidates scoring more than two marks. Gonorrhoea and syphilis were the most commonly offered answers.

 *Pitfall: No-one added the term **primary** syphilis, which is relevant to the stem as it asked for diseases suggesting recent sexual encounters.*

The other answers included candidiasis, chlamydia, herpes, hepatitis and HIV. Candida is not a notifiable disease. The others may be subclinical for some time and therefore cannot be used for accurate dating, e.g. as in rape cases, or can be contracted in other ways.

	Score
B► 1. False	1
2. False	1
3. True	1
4. False	1

1.   Very disappointing. Only one candidate was correct.

2 & 3. Over two thirds of the candidates had the right answers for these two questions.

 Howler!

*4. Surprisingly, only half the candidates were aware that gonorrhoea could not be isolated from a high vaginal swab. Neisseria gonorrhoeae is a delicate organism, requiring prompt plating to grow. It is isolated from endocervical, urethral, throat and rectal swabs but **not** high vaginal swabs. Bartholin's abscesses can be associated and swabs should always be sent at the time of incision and drainage. The prevalence of penicillin-resistant strains of gonorrhoea is 10%. The standard treatment is a STAT dose of oral ciprofloxacin.*

ANSWERS/COMMENTS

Score

C➤ Contact tracing, to offer diagnostic screening and treatment 1

Most candidates were correct although several quoted 'treat the partner'. Often there is more than one partner involved and 'contact tracing' is a better term to use as it covers all eventualities.

Some candidates thought that sex education and advice regarding safe sex was the answer. This is important, of course, but the stem did have a hint of urgency in the wording 'vitally important' and contact tracing is the more immediate priority.

D➤ The use of the oral contraceptive pill, which offers efficient contraception, with the sheath or cap, as a protection against sexually transmitted disease 1

Unbelievably, very few candidates were familiar with this very commonly used family planning term, especially relevant to Young People's Clinics (formerly Youth Advisory Services).

 Howler! Sharing the bill at the end of your meal.

This question has been written in conjunction with a genitourinary consultant.

STRUCTURED ORAL

Instructions to candidate

A 55-year-old lady attends your surgery for advice regarding HRT. She is oligomenorrhoeic; her last period was four months ago. Her initial vasomotor symptoms have settled, but she complains of tiredness, aches and pains, generalized pruritus, vaginal dryness and loss of libido. She smokes 15 cigarettes per day but has no other medical problems. There is a strong family history of ischaemic heart disease but nil else of note.

Please discuss your management of this with the examiner.

Instructions to examiner

You will need to discuss the management of this case with the candidate.

A➤ The lady is interested in 'no bleed' preparations.

1. What would you do to decide if she is a suitable candidate for this form of HRT?

2. Name two different types of 'no bleed' hormone replacement regimes.

3. In counselling this patient, what is the main disadvantage you should bring to her attention?

4. How else might you assist her lack of libido?

B➤ She is worried about the risks of breast cancer on HRT. What information and advice would you give her (maximum two marks to be awarded for well-balanced argument).

C➤ She has read recently that some new studies have reported an increased incidence of thrombosis on HRT.

1. How great is the risk? Put the data into perspective for her (allow two marks for detailed answer, one mark for basic facts).

2. In the light of these facts, how would you modify your prescribing habits?

ANSWERS/COMMENTS

	Score

A➤ 1. Ultrasound scan to check endometrial thickness/does the
endometrium look inactive? Progestogen challenge test. (No
withdrawal bleed indicates inactive endometrium.) ... **1**

    2. a A gonadomimetic, e.g. tibolone ... **1**

       b Continuous combined therapy (CCT) ... **1**

    3. On CCT there is a 30% chance of initial breakthrough bleeding (in ... **1**
60–80% of cases breakthrough bleeding has ceased within six
months). There is some risk of irregular bleeding with tibolone but it
is less (usually first 2–3 cycles only). ... **1**

    4. Testosterone implants
Vaginal creams
Counselling

1. The majority of the candidates were far too general in their
approach to this question. They were asked specifically what they
would do to decide if the patient were suitable for 'this form of
HRT', i.e. a 'no bleed' preparation. In the main, answers addressed
the need for a general assessment of the patient, i.e. blood pressure, menopausal status, current FSH level, previous thrombosis.

2. Again, candidates were asked to name two different types of
preparation, not two different preparations. The majority quoted
different brands initially. With prompting, most offered either
tibolone or a continuous combined preparation; only 30% of candidates offered both. There seemed to be a general confusion that
tibolone was a different approach, i.e. a gonadomimetic rather
than continuous oestrogen and continuous progestogen combined.

3. Only half the candidates appreciated the need to counsel patients
on the risk of initial bleedings with these preparations. This is a
potent cause of non-compliance. Women who opt for a preparation to avoid bleeds get quickly disillusioned if breakthrough
bleeding occurs. A realistic assessment of how likely this is to occur
and for how long before prescribing will help them to persevere.

4. Genuine loss of libido usually requires testosterone. Loss of confidence / vaginismus secondary to superficial dyspareunia may well
be helped with topical oestrogens. Atrophic vaginitis causes sore-
ness, dryness and irritation. It can also cause contact bleeding if
severe.

ANSWERS/COMMENTS

Score

B➤ Two extra cases of breast cancer per 1000 women on HRT for five years. Six extra cases of breast cancer per 1000 women on HRT for ten years.

1–2

Risks to be balanced against advantages at this stage; she has increased risk of ischaemic heart disease – smoker and strong family history. Estimated 35% reduction in mortality from IHD in HRT users.

The majority of candidates made a credible attempt at this complex issue in the short time allowed, but then time is pressing in a busy general practice surgery and it is important to have the ability to put information across clearly and concisely.

C➤ 1. Estimated 2–4-fold increased risk. In real terms, this means instead of a background baseline risk of 1 in 10 000, in HRT users the risk is 3 in 10 000 per year (the Oxford study quotes 1 per 5000, the Harvard study quotes 1 per 10 000). Mortality is approximately 1–2% in thrombosis cases, plus the risk of thromboembolism seems to disappear after HRT stops. The risk is the same for all types of HRT and all oestrogen doses. The risk is highest in the first year.

1–2

2. Exclude women with high risk of thrombosis from HRT, i.e. personal or family history of thromboembolism, severe varicose veins, obesity, prolonged bed rest, surgery, trauma. Overall, the small risk does not outweigh the considerable benefits of HRT – women without predisposing factors need not stop taking it.

1

The risk of thrombosis in HRT users was accurately quoted and most candidates were able to see this issue in perspective and counsel accordingly. There was a reluctance to prescribe HRT in previous thrombosis sufferers or in those with a family history. There was little understanding of the concept of thrombophilia screening (see Circuit E Station 5 answers.)

QUESTIONS

The modern management of ectopic pregnancies has changed with better investigative and surgical techniques available.

A➤ What level of sensitivity does the β-hCG urine test offer?

B➤ At what week gestation can a foetal heart be detected:

1. on an abdominal probe ultrasound?

2. on a vaginal probe ultrasound?

C➤ Given that the urinary pregnancy test is positive but the ultrasound showed an empty uterine cavity and you are monitoring the patient by serial β-hCG levels:

1. What is the normal rise of serum β-hCG in pregnancy?

2. At what level would you decide that a laparoscopy was indicated?

D➤ Many units are now performing laparoscopic salpingotomy instead of open surgery. List three advantages to the patient.

1.

2.

3.

E➤ 1. What is the tubal patency rate after laparoscopic salpingotomy?

2. Is the intrauterine pregnancy rate higher after laparoscopic or formal salpingotomy?

ANSWERS/COMMENTS

Score

A► **Sensitivity greater than 50 iu**
1

There was considerable confusion here. Many candidates obviously were thinking of sensitivity and specificity and therefore quoted their answers in percentages. For pregnancy tests, however, it is common to quote the level of β-hCG the test would detect in international units.

B► 1. 6–7 weeks
1

2. 5–6 weeks
1

The majority of candidates were aware that abdominal probe scanning was less sensitive than vaginal scanning. Some candidates thought that it would be eight weeks before an abdominal scan could detect a foetal heart.

C► 1. β-hCG doubles in 48 hours
1

2. Greater than 1000 iu
1

Many candidates felt the decision to perform laparoscopy should be based on a trend of rising β-hCG and clinical signs. This is too non-specific. The question had a detailed stem, quoting an empty uterine cavity on scan and asking specifically for the level of β-hCG at which laparoscopy should be performed, if serial monitoring was occurring.

 Differentiator: Approximately one third of candidates were correct for each part. Some thought the levels doubled in a week or quoted a steady linear rise, i.e. 30 iu per week.

D► **Any three of the following:**
3

1. The patient has smaller scars
2. Better cosmetic results
3. Less analgesia required
4. Patient is discharged home from hospital on day 2
5. Patient can return to work after 2–3 weeks
6. Less chance of pelvic adhesions
7. More chance of future conception

A good attempt by most candidates. The majority were correct for two out of three answers. 'More chance of saving the tube' was an irrelevant answer since a salpingotomy was the operation quoted, whether done at laparoscopy or laparotomy.

ANSWERS/COMMENTS

E➤ 1. 70%   1

2. Laparoscopic salpingotomy   1

Most candidates were in the range of 60–80% for the tubal patency rate and over 90% agreed that the intrauterine pregnancy rate was higher after laparoscopic surgery.

Circuit D

QUESTIONS

A woman attends your surgery at 26 weeks' gestation in her second pregnancy. Her first baby was delivered by emergency caesarean section as a result of foetal distress following a scalp pH of 7.14. The cervix at that time was dilated to 6 cm. At today's visit the symphyseal fundal height corresponds to her menstrual dates and the presentation is cephalic.

A► She is keen to have an idea of what her chances of vaginal delivery might be this time. What figure would you tell her?

_____ %

B► What is the main risk associated with a trial of labour in this lady's case?

_____

C► What form of antenatal care would you consider appropriate: shared care, modified shared care or full hospital care?

_____

D► What three initial separate steps would you take as the SHO admitting this patient in established labour?

1. _____

2. _____

3. _____

E► List four classic signs of the problem in question B.

1. _____

2. _____

3. _____

4. _____

ANSWERS/COMMENTS

Score

A➤ 70–80%

1

Only a third of candidates have given an accurate assessment. This is essential information to allow you to counsel your patients.

B➤ Rupture of the uterus

1

 Howlers! Most candidates got this right, but a few howlers have been presented – cephalopelvic disproportion; placental abruption.

C➤ Shared care

1

The point of this question is that this lady will require extra supervision in labour but she may be booked for shared antenatal care. The term 'modified shared care' has caused some confusion. It is used to describe those situations where more of the antenatal care is undertaken in hospital but the mother still sees the community midwife and GP, for example twin pregnancies which need to come to hospital for growth scans.

D➤ Any three of the following:

3

1. Set up an intravenous access.
2. Send blood for group and crossmatch.
3. Inform the registrar of the case.
4. Establish continuous cardiotocographic monitoring.

This section caused a lot of controversy. Many candidates wanted to examine the lady as a priority. Given that there is a previous caesarean scar present, it is reasonable to defer examination until after assessing the foetus, establishing intravenous access and contacting more senior personnel.

 Howler! Introduce yourself.

ANSWERS/COMMENTS

E➤ Any four of the following:

1. Foetal distress
2. Heavy vaginal bleeding
3. Frank haematuria
4. Absence of presenting part in the pelvis on vaginal examination
5. Continual pain (breaking through epidural analgesia
6. Ill-defined suprapubic swelling/foetal parts more easily palpable abdominally
7. Shock

Obviously, candidates had to get question B correct to enable them to answer this part. A number of candidates suggested a fall in blood pressure, rapid pulse and pallor as separate signs. The examiner would only accept one of these as they are all symptomatic of shock.

QUESTIONS

The main reason for the dramatic fall in the incidence of rhesus disease is the administration of anti-D immunoglobulin to rhesus-negative mothers.

A► List two features in a primiparous mother's history at booking which might alert you to an increased risk of rhesus disease in the foetus.

1.

2.

B► List five situations in which anti-D immunoglobulin should be given to a rhesus-negative mother.

1.

2.

3.

4.

5.

C► What is the Kleihauer test?

D► You are called to see a woman at home who is 13 weeks pregnant with vaginal bleeding. Assessing the situation, you are happy for her to rest at home. She is rhesus negative.

1. What dose of anti-D immunoglobulin would you administer?

2. Within what time limit of the start of her bleeding must it be given to be effective?

ANSWERS/COMMENTS

	Score

A➤ 1. Previous transfusion   **1**

     2. Threatened miscarriage   **1**

Many candidates have suggested rhesus-negative mother but this is in the stem and therefore will not be accepted. Others have suggested previous antepartum haemorrhage termination, miscarriages, etc. but the stem said 'primiparous'. Read the question!

B➤ Any five of the following: **5**

    1. Miscarriage   5. External cephalic version

    2. Termination   6. Intrauterine transfusion

    3. Amniocentesis   7. Antepartum haemorrhage

    4. Cordocentesis   8. Following delivery in a rhesus-negative mother

Quite a list, so candidates should be able to give six. In some units it is routinely given to primiparous rhesus-negative mothers at 28 and 34 weeks.

C➤ Measures the quantity of foetal blood that enters the maternal circulation   **1**

 Howlers! A test to detect rhesus antibodies in the mother; test using foetal blood to estimate the presence of antibodies.

500 iu anti-D immunoglobulin can eliminate up to 4.0 ml of Rh-D negative blood from the maternal circulation. If there is a possibility of greater sensitization, for example, delivery after 20 weeks' gestation or placental abruption, a Kleihauer test should be performed to see if extra anti-D immunoglobulin is required.

D➤ 1. 250 international units/litre   **1**

     2. 72 hours   **1**

Only 65% of candidates have answered correctly. Answers ranged from 50 to 1200 units. This is vital information for a GP who will look after women with threatened miscarriages at home. The continued occurrence of rhesus isoimmunization is due in part to the failure to give any or enough anti-D when indicated. The second reason is that sensitization can occur during the first pregnancy in the absence of any complication. This may occur in up to 2% of rhesus-negative primigravidae. It is because of this that some units give a routine injection of 250 iu anti-D immunoglobulin at 28 and 34 weeks. The cost-effectiveness of this measure is still uncertain, but we did accept it as an answer to B.

QUESTIONS

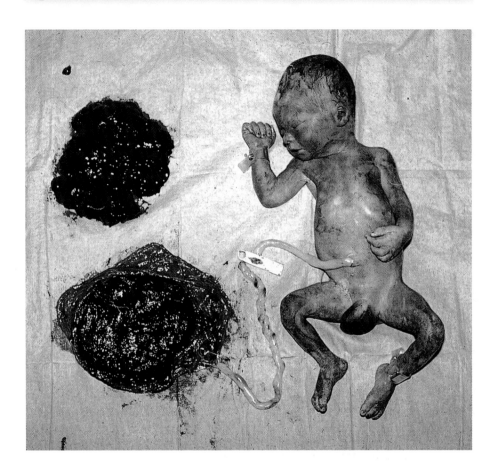

QUESTIONS

A► What does the photograph demonstrate?

_____

B► Give three factors that may have contributed to the primary condition.

1. _____

2. _____

3. _____

C► List three steps in the immediate management of the mother's acute presenting condition.

1. _____

2. _____

3. _____

D► List two maternal complications of this condition.

1. _____

2. _____

E► What is the risk of this clinical condition recurring in her next pregnancy?

_____

ANSWERS/COMMENTS

Score

A➤ Placental abruption, intrauterine death

1

Forty-eight percent of candidates have given both components of the answer. Intrauterine death or abruption alone is not a complete answer.

B➤ Any three of the following:

3

1. Trauma
2. Uterine distension
3. Grand multiparity
4. Pregnancy-induced hypertension
5. Smoking
6. External cephalic version

The majority of candidates have scored two marks here. There was confusion between high parity and increasing maternal age. One can be of high parity and still be young, hence maternal age alone is not an acceptable answer. A number of candidates have offered diabetes. While this can lead to polyhydramnios, it is too removed from the problem to be an acceptable answer. Placenta praevia, mentioned by some candidates, is not associated with placental abruption.

C➤ Any three of the following:

3

1. Establish intravenous access in the mother.
2. Resuscitate if necessary.
3. Group and crossmatch mother's blood.
4. Check mother's blood for level of clotting factors.
5. Expedite delivery of the foetus.

Many candidates have fallen into the trap of discussing bereavement management. We are looking for the acute management of this life-threatening condition. Candidates have complained that they did not offer delivery as an answer because the photograph showed a dead baby, yet one may need to perform a section for an intrauterine death if the cervix is unfavourable and early disseminated intravascular coagulation occurs.

ANSWERS/COMMENTS

	Score

D➤ Any two of the following: 2

1. Disseminated intravascular coagulopathy
2. Renal failure
3. Adult respiratory distress syndrome
4. Hypovolaemic shock
5. Postpartum haemorrhage

Most candidates have managed to give two correct answers.

E➤ 5–8% 1

This has been poorly answered; most candidates said 1–2%.

QUESTIONS

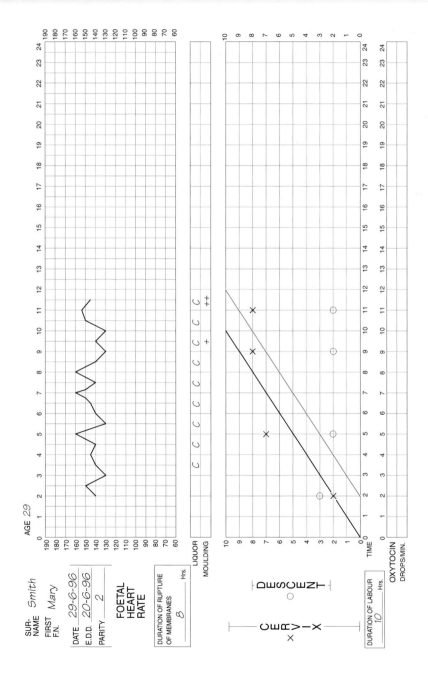

AGE *29*

SUR- *Smith*
NAME

FIRST *Mary*
F.N.

DATE *29-6-96*
E.D.D. *20-6-96*
PARITY *2*

FOETAL
HEART
RATE

DURATION OF RUPTURE
OF MEMBRANES _____ *8* _____ Hrs.

LIQUOR

MOULDING

D E S C E N T

C E R V I X

TIME

DURATION OF LABOUR
_____ *10* _____ Hrs.

OXYTOCIN

DROPS/MIN.

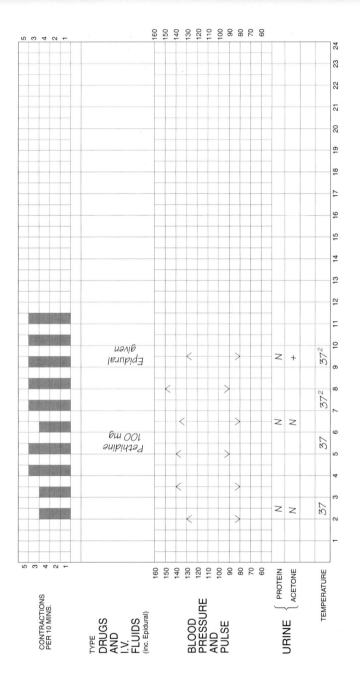

QUESTIONS

The partogram illustrates the progress of a 29-year-old multiparous lady. Her first baby weighed 3.2 kg and was delivered by Neville Barnes forceps. The second baby was a spontaneous vaginal delivery, at term, weighing 3.9 kg.

A➤ What does this partogram show?

B➤ List three different clinical situations in which this could occur.

1.

2.

3.

C➤ What is the principal risk to this mother?

D➤ How would you manage this lady?

1. Commence syntocinon.

   Yes/No

2. Reassess progress in two hours.

   Yes/No

3. Expedite delivery by Ventouse.

   Yes/No

4. Deliver by caesarean section.

   Yes/No

5. Insert an intrauterine pressure catheter.

   Yes/No

ANSWERS/COMMENTS

Score

A► **Secondary arrest (at 8 cm with high head at station 2)** | 1

In validation, only 27% of candidates provided the correct answer. Most answers were too non-specific, such as: uterine dysfunction, poor progress in the first stage.

B► 1. Cephalopelvic disproportion | 1
2. Malpresentation – face, brow | 1
3. Malposition – occipitoposterior, deep transverse arrest | 1

This section was handled very badly at validation. Only 8% of candidates gave the correct answer to all three parts.

 Tip: Many answered 'diabetes' or 'big baby'. These are insufficient answers alone. Diabetes may lead to a large baby but whether it will deliver vaginally depends on the size of the pelvis.

 Howlers! Cervical stenosis; full bladder; maternal ketoacidosis and immobility.

C► **Rupture of the uterus** | 1

At validation, only 40% of answers were correct. This demonstrates a lack of basic knowledge about the main risk of obstructed labour in a multiparous woman.

D► 1. No | 1
2. No | 1
3. No | 1
4. Yes | 1
5. No | 1

In general, this has been answered poorly. The partogram shows that this woman has made good progress to 8 cm with good contractions. Delivery by caesarean section is the best course of action. Insertion of an intrauterine pressure catheter might be considered by some experienced obstetricians to see if the uterine contractions are adequate. We felt this, therefore, might be regarded as a controversial question, but in fact 81% of candidates scored a mark for answering 'No'.

QUESTIONS

John and Mary attend your surgery to discuss sterilization. John is aged 36 and Mary 29. They have three children aged six, four and 18 months, all of whom are well. Mary is a diabetic and therefore they feel John should be the one to be sterilized.

A► List three advantages of male sterilization.

1.

2.

3.

B► How long will John need to be off work if:

1. he is an office worker?

2. he does heavy manual work?

C► How will you confirm that the procedure is effective?

D► List two short-term complications.

1.

2.

E► What advice might be given to reduce these two short-term complications?

1.

2.

ANSWERS/COMMENTS

	Score

A▶ Any three from the following: **3**

1. Performed under local anaesthetic
2. Significant operation morbidity and mortality are virtually non-existent
3. Easy procedure to perform
4. Cheaper (less sophisticated equipment than female sterilization)
5. Usually involves less disruption to family than female sterilization
6. No inpatient stay

General practitioners need to have some knowledge of male steriliza-tion techniques and certainly to be able to accurately present the advantages and disadvantages of male versus female sterilization when counselling patients.

 Howlers! There are several possible answers to choose from here and really all candidates should have earned three marks without much effort. However, there have been howlers, e.g. 'A GA may be necessary'.

B▶ 1. Just the day of the procedure **1**
2. Two or three days **1**

The answers to this have been widely divergent.

 Howlers! Many candidates have felt that even if John is an office worker he would need to take two weeks off work and if he is per-forming heavy manual labour anything from six weeks to three months off work.

C▶ Negative seminal analysis 12 and 16 weeks after the vasectomy **1**

Here, 50% of the candidates have given the correct number of semen analyses to be performed, i.e. two or three, but did not offer any time scale. The other 50% have guessed that some form of assessment would be necessary at 12 weeks but did not comment that two con-secutive semen analyses were needed.

 Differentiator: In fact, only 10% of the candidates have been total-ly correct for this question.

ANSWERS/COMMENTS

	Score

D➤ 1. Scrotal haematoma or bleeding   1

2. Wound infection or epididymitis   1

Some very interesting answers have been given regarding short-term complications.

The majority of candidates have been correct but it is important to remember that failure of the procedure is not a *short-term* complication. Fifteen percent of candidates have offered pain as an option; this is a little non-specific. Moreover, severe pain would be secondary to haematoma or infection.

E➤ Any two of the following: 2

1. Wear a good, firm scrotal support, night and day for the first two weeks.
2. Maintain good hygiene.
3. Sexual activity may be resumed as soon as there is no further discomfort.

Several candidates have offered advice such as 'good hygiene' or 'avoid exercise and weight lifting'. We had not previously intended to include good hygiene as one of these acceptable answers but it is basic common sense to tell patients this and therefore we have added it to our answer pool.

QUESTIONS

During surgery one morning, the receptionist asks you to take a telephone call from Mr Brown who is ringing you about his wife who is 38 weeks pregnant. He is clearly very concerned that his wife has developed quite severe abdominal pain and is having to lie down as she feels lightheaded. This is her fifth pregnancy and you had seen her earlier the previous day in your antenatal clinic, looking very well.

A➤ Which of the following would be most appropriate?

1. Advise he waits till her lightheadedness improves then brings her round to the surgery in his car (they live just around the corner).

   Yes/No

2. Take her direct to the nearest casualty.

   Yes/No

3. Bring his wife straight to the surgery.

   Yes/No

4. Dial 999 for an ambulance.

   Yes/No

5. Visit the patient after surgery to assess the situation and manage as appropriate.

   Yes/No

B➤ What are the two most important tests you would like to perform on admission to determine the diagnosis?

1.

2.

C➤ List three recognized complications of grand multiparity.

1.

2.

3.

ANSWERS/COMMENTS

Score

A➤ 1. No   1
    2. No   1
    3. No   1
    4. Yes   1
    5. No   1

In validation, only 35% of candidates answered this question correctly.

The Royal College of Anaesthetists has mandatory stations that must be answered correctly in order to pass the examination, whilst the Royal College of Obstetricians and Gynaecologists does not do this as yet. This type of station, which tests basic obstetric emergency management, could easily be regarded as a mandatory station. It was written by a GP tutor, not an obstetrician.

B➤ 1. Ultrasound scan   1
    2. Midstream urine for culture   1

In validation, most candidates suggested maternal examination, including blood pressure.

 Pitfall: These are not tests – read the question.

Again, most wished to perform a cardiotocograph, but the question asked for tests to determine the diagnosis, not to assess the baby.

C➤ Any three of the following: 3

    1. Precipitous labour
    2. Unstable lie/cord prolapse
    3. Uterine rupture
    4. Postpartum haemorrhage
    5. Maternal anaemia
    6. Abruption

Performance in this question was generally good. Grand multiparity does not necessarily mean the mother is elderly, therefore pregnancy-induced hypertension and diabetes (complications of age) are not accepted. Maternal anaemia is accepted but will usually occur only if the pregnancies are close together.

 Howlers! Failure to progress; preterm labour.

Wendy is 33 years of age and four weeks postdelivery of her fourth child. The pregnancy had been uncomplicated and Daniel, her son, was born at term as a normal vaginal delivery.

Your attached midwife telephones you and asks you to visit because Wendy has passed a large clot (the previous day) and continues to bleed.

A➤ List five facts that you would need to assess to determine the urgency of the case.

1.

2.

3.

4.

5.

B➤ What two important features would you elicit on vaginal examination to confirm a diagnosis?

1.

2.

C➤ In this particular case, what is the most likely cause of bleeding?

D➤ What other cause could be implicated?

E➤ What simple fact would make your answer to D unlikely?

ANSWERS/COMMENTS

Score

A➤ Any five of the following: **5**

1. Blood pressure
2. Pulse
3. Shocked/pale/sweating/general appearance
4. Estimated blood loss
5. Abdominal pain
6. Uterine size
7. Uterine tenderness

This question is designed to test if candidates can evaluate the *degree of urgency* over the telephone. Questions about bleeding patterns postdelivery or associated smelly discharge will not help assess the degree of urgency, though they may need to be asked later. Again, this station was vetted by a GP tutor.

 Howler! Does Wendy live alone, in a remote place with no phone!

B➤ 1. Is the cervical os open or closed?   **1**
      2. Is uterine size compatible with normal rate of involution?   **1**

You need to exclude the presence of retained products of conception which would require Wendy to be referred to hospital.

Many candidates have answered 'tenderness' but this is not one of the most important features. It is non-specific and does not allow a diagnosis to be made.

C➤ Retained products of conception   **1**

This question has been answered well. Some candidates queried infection, considering four weeks postpartum to be too long for retained products. Usually the stem would be more specific, commenting on pyrexia, rigours or offensive discharge.

 Howler! Multiparity. This is associated with postpartum haemorrhage, not bleeding one month postdelivery.

D➤ Having a period   **1**

Only 35% of candidates have suggested the correct answer. Maybe they felt four weeks was too soon to have a period, but it is much more likely than some of the proposed answers: endometriosis, gestational trophoblastic disease.

ANSWERS/COMMENTS

	Score
E➤ If she was breast feeding	**1**

Candidates have struggled here because they did not know the answer to D. This was designed to make candidates think laterally.

QUESTIONS

Score

Mrs Smith is 37 years old and has just presented at your surgery antenatal clinic ten weeks pregnant. She is very concerned about her risk of having a Down syndrome baby.

A► What would you estimate her risk to be, based on her age alone?

B► What two important factors in her past history would significantly increase this risk?

1.

2.

C► In counselling this patient before embarking on amniocentesis:

1. Name two widely available tests which would further determine her risk factor other than her age alone.

a

b

2. At what stage in pregnancy is each of these routinely performed?

D► 1. What further test is currently being evaluated as a Down marker?

2. What advantage does this test offer over the others?

QUESTIONS

E➤ What single specific piece of advice would you give this lady about the interpretation of these results?

F➤ If Mrs Smith opts for an amniocentesis, what is her risk of miscarriage following the procedure if it is performed at 15 weeks' gestation?

%

ANSWERS/COMMENTS

	Score

A➤ 1:190 to 1:250 (dependent on age at delivery) — 1

The ability to counsel a woman about the risk of Down syndrome is an essential element of general practice. We would expect candidates to have a figure for the risk at 37 years of age. A generous range is given yet less than 50% of candidates were correct.

B➤ 1. Family history — 1
2. Previous Down baby — 1

The majority of candidates have suggested a previous affected child. A family history is very important, allowing you to test parental chromosomes and potentially avoid invasive testing on the foetus.

C➤ 1. a Maternal α-fetoprotein — 1
   b Leeds/Barts/triple test — 1
2. 14–18 weeks — 1

The key word in this question is *widely*, which means only serum testing is acceptable. A number of candidates have suggested ultrasound but this is too non-specific. There are specific ultrasound markers for Down syndrome but not every affected foetus has them. The 'soft' markers for Down syndrome are:

- choroid plexus cysts
- pyelectasis
- ventricular 'golf balls'
- short femur
- nuchal fold.

If any of these is detected, amniocentesis is offered. Some candidates were critical of the answer 'maternal serum α-fetoprotein (AFP), considering this to be an old-fashioned test no longer widely used. However, the examination has to reflect clinical trends *nationally* and this test is still used extensively. Low maternal serum AFP (2.5 SD < normal) will indicate increased risk of Down syndrome. High maternal serum AFP alone will detect the majority of open neural tube defects, 90% of anencephalic foetuses and 80% of spina bifida foetuses. The national incidence of neural tube defects ranges between three and eight per 1000 births.

For information on the triple test, which increases the accuracy for risk assessment, see comments on Circuit B, Station 8.

 Tip: Amniocentesis and chorionic villus sampling offer diagnosis. The question asked for 'tests' to determine 'risk factor'. Read the question!

ANSWERS/COMMENTS

	Score
D► 1. Nuchal fold thickness	1
2. Can be done at 11 weeks	1

Nuchal fold screening has the advantage of being performed at an earlier gestation. If a mother has a high risk of a Down baby she can be offered chorionic villus sampling.

The original work on nuchal fold thickness was performed on high-risk groups. The thickness is proportional to the gestational age. Thus, this must be standardized between centres. The best time to perform nuchal fold thickness is at 11 weeks' gestation. Further work is currently being carried out, hence the careful phrasing of the stem to D.1, 'currently being evaluated as a Down marker'.

 Tip: If you offered nuchal fold screening for one of the answers in C.1 you should go back and think again. It is highly unlikely that two questions at a station will have the same answer.

E► **These tests only offer a probability, not a definite diagnosis.**   1

F► **1%**   1

Only 53% of candidates have answered this question correctly but this is basic information needed when counselling women. Many quoted a rate of 2%.

REST STATION

STRUCTURED ORAL

Score

Instructions to candidate

Mrs Poultney has had recurrent problems with a bad back ever since she suffered a slipped disc four years ago. She had a difficult time with her first pregnancy and did not want an epidural in labour. The pethidine she was given made her drowsy and nauseated without providing adequate analgesia. At 6 cm dilation of her cervix, she capitulated and had an epidural. Sadly, after delivery she experienced backache and a bad headache.

She is now pregnant for the second time and has come to discuss analgesia for her forthcoming labour.

Instructions to examiner

You play the role of Mrs Poultney who has had recurrent problems with a bad back ever since a slipped disc four years ago.

She had a difficult time with her first pregnancy and did not want an epidural in labour. However, pethidine made her drowsy and nauseated without providing adequate analgesia. At 6 cm she capitulated and had an epidural. Sadly, she had a bad headache and backache afterwards.

She is now pregnant for the second time and has come to discuss analgesia for her forthcoming labour.

Please ensure that you lead the candidate through all the following questions in the time allocated.

A➤ I am very concerned, Doctor. After all, I was in labour for 13 hours last time and the pain was very bad at the end. What can I expect my second delivery to be like?

B➤ I would like to stay as mobile as possible in labour. Can you give me some facts about the new mobile epidural? What is it? How does it work?

1. _____

2. _____

C➤ Are there any problems associated with the new mobile epidural? (Please prompt the candidate – they must mention three problems.)

1. _____

2. _____

3. _____

STRUCTURED ORAL

Score

D➤ How effective is the new mobile epidural in terms of pain relief?

E➤ Is it suitable for everyone, Doctor? How would you decide who should be offered a mobile epidural? (You are looking for three criteria here.)

1. _____

2. _____

3. _____

ANSWERS/COMMENTS

	Score

A➤ Needs an explanation that the second labour is usually shorter and easier whatever analgesia is chosen. Average duration of labour in a multiparous patient is eight hours. (If the second baby is substantially larger than the first, progress in labour would be modified.) — **1**

B➤ 1. A combined spinal/epidural (CSE) technique using a weak solution of local anaesthetic with a small dose of short-acting opiate. — **1**

2. The spinal provides early analgesia. — **1**

C➤ 1. Difficult to assess the upper level of the block (implications if emergency caesarean section is ultimately needed). — **1**

2. Some breakthrough pain is possible. — **1**

3. After several 'top ups' most women find they are no longer ambulatory. — **1**

D➤ Not 100% effective in all patients. Probably 100% effective in approximately 70% of patients. — **1**

E➤ 1. Patient must be well motivated and *want* to be mobile. — **1**

2. There should always be someone readily available when the patient is walking (in case she stumbles or falls) so that the partner (relative or friend) must be well motivated to assist and must be available for support throughout labour. — **1**

3. An understanding of the technique and its limitations is important, therefore a poor command of English, or lack of interpreter with fluent English, is a relative contraindication. — **1**

This station has been answered poorly by most of the candidates. Range of marks 0–9, mean 4.6, standard deviation 2.0.

Those candidates who have been good were very good indeed. Some candidates displayed a knowledge of epidurals in general but not mobile epidurals in particular.

Although an in-depth knowledge is not expected, general practitioners must obviously keep up to date with new techniques, particularly regarding analgesia in labour. This is something that all patients will want to know about.

QUESTIONS

One of your routine visits today is to Mrs Peters for a postnatal visit. Her only complaints are an offensive vaginal discharge and constipation. Study the attached maternal discharge summary.

A➤ What two factors may have contributed to this lady's discharge?

1. _____

2. _____

B➤ List two reasons why this lady might be constipated.

1. _____

2. _____

C➤ The investigations which you now feel are required are:

1. full blood count.

   Yes/No _____

2. high vaginal swab.

   Yes/No _____

3. ultrasound.

   Yes/No _____

4. smear.

   Yes/No _____

D➤ What specific concern would you have in assessing the baby both now and at subsequent developmental assessments?

_____

_____

E➤ What review arrangements will you make for the baby?

_____

QUESTIONS

MATERNITY UNIT
MOTHER AND BABY DISCHARGE SUMMARY

Mrs Peters
Date of discharge: 11.06.96

LABOUR AND DELIVERY

Time and date of delivery	*23.09 hr on 08.06.96*
Onset of labour	*Spontaneous*
Duration of labour	*12 hours 50 minutes*
Analgesia	*Epidural*
Mode of delivery	*Low forceps*
Perineum	*Episiotomy*
Complications	*Meconium liquor. Ragged membranes*

PUERPERIUM

Haemoglobin	*9.8 g/dl*
Anti-D	*Not required*
Rubella vaccination	*Not required*
Proposed contraception	*Progesterone-only pill*
Discharge medication	*Ferrous sulphate – one a day*

BABY'S DETAILS

Sex	*Male*
Gestation	*41 weeks 4 days*
APGAR	*06–10*
Birth head circumference	*35 cm*
Weight at birth	*3460 grams*
Feeding at discharge	*Breast*
Cord	*Not separated*
Guthrie	*Not done*
BCG immunisation	*Not given*
Congenital abnormalities	*None*
Complications	*Mild meconium aspiration treated with gentamicin*

Follow-up

ANSWERS/COMMENTS

	Score
A► 1. Retained products of conception/endometritis	1
2. Infected episiotomy	1

In validation, only 30% of candidates scored both marks. Answers like infection or instrumental delivery are too non-specific.

B► 1. Iron therapy — 1
2. Painful perineum — 1

 Tip: *You will only score marks if the answers you give relate to the discharge summary. For example, some candidates have answered 'piles', which could lead to constipation, but piles do not appear on the summary.*

 Howler! *Large uterus pressing on the bowel.*

C► 1. Yes — 1
2. Yes — 1
3. No — 1
4. No — 1

Almost 50% of candidates would request an ultrasound. It is usually unhelpful in these circumstances. The report will nearly always comment on the presence of blood clot in the uterus. This is not significant. It is far more important to exclude infection in Mrs Peters' case.

D► Its hearing — 1

This question has been very badly answered. The question asked for a *specific* concern. The discharge summary stated that the baby had been treated with gentamicin.

 Tip: *If you offer two answers (as many candidates have), only the first is marked even if the second is correct.*

 Howlers! *Is the baby feeding well? Neonatal infection.*

A few candidates offered facial palsy secondary to the forceps delivery. If this had occurred it would have appeared in the discharge summary.

ANSWERS/COMMENTS

E➤ Formal hearing test at eight months

Sadly, if you got D wrong you also lost the marks for E.

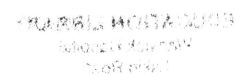

QUESTIONS

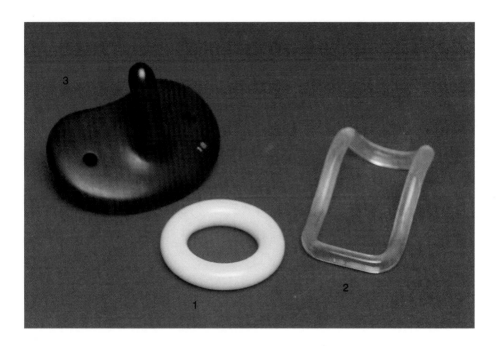

QUESTIONS

Score

A▶ Identify the three structures in front of you.

1. _____

2. _____

3. _____

B▶ What is the function of:

1. structure 1?

   _____

2. structure 2?

   _____

C▶ Consider structure 1.

1. How often should it be changed?

   _____

2. List four possible complications of usage.

   a _____

   b _____

   c _____

   d _____

ANSWERS/COMMENTS

	Score

A➤ 1. Ring pessary ... 1
2. Hodge pessary ... 1
3. Shelf pessary ... 1

A third of the candidates identified all three structures correctly.

> **Howlers!**
> Item 2: *gadget for improving the strength of the pelvic floor.*
> Item 3: *many candidates felt this was a 'vaginal dilator'.*

B➤ 1. Uterovaginal prolapse ... 1
2. Correcting a retroverted uterus ... 1

While 70% knew the function of a ring pessary, almost nobody gave the correct function of a Hodge pessary, which is to antevert a retro-verted uterus. It is not that commonly used. The principal indication is deep dyspareunia associated with retroversion. In many of these cases, however, the retroversion is fixed by adhesions. It can also be used in early pregnancy if a retroverted uterus causes urinary retention.

C➤ 1. Six-monthly ... 1

> **Howler!** *Three years.*

2. Any four of the following: ... 4
  a Bleeding
  b Vaginal discharge/infection
  c Faecal impaction
  d Urinary retention
  e Inability to retain pessary

Quite a wide range here but in the main well answered.

Bleeding usually results from pressure on atrophic vaginal skin. The vaginal skin should be inspected each time the ring is changed. If it is excoriated or ulcerated the ring should be left out and topical oestro-gen prescribed daily for 2–4 weeks. If still ulcerated, the patient should be referred for biopsy. Some older patients who are unable to insert the oestrogen cream themselves may need daily district nurse visits or admission for oestrogen-coated vaginal pack and catheter for 1–2 weeks. Too large a ring may cause urinary retention or faecal impaction.

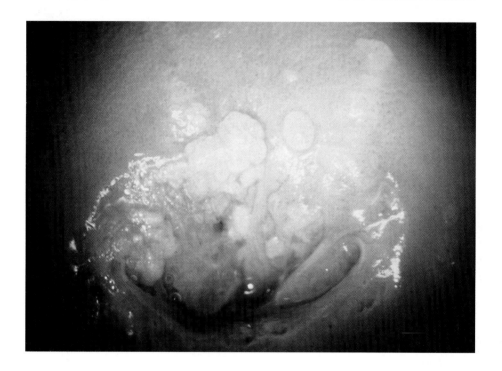

QUESTIONS

Score

A➤ Which is the most common sexually transmitted disease?

_____

B➤ If *Chlamydia trachomatis* is isolated from an endocervical swab:

1. a singe dose of tetracycline is adequate treatment preoperatively for termination of pregnancy.

True/False
_____

2. risk of infection is enhanced in the presence of atopy.

True/False
_____

3. long-term complications may be mediated by a host-determined immune response.

True/False
_____

C➤ Name three long-term complications of *Chlamydia trachomatis* infection.

1. _____

2. _____

3. _____

D➤ Study the photograph in front of you.

1. What does it show?

_____

2. In which condition has it been implicated as an aetiological factor?

_____

E➤ Name one other factor predisposing to this condition.

_____

ANSWERS/COMMENTS

Score

A➤ Genital wart virus infection

1

This question has been answered very poorly. Most candidates have offered *Chlamydia* which is the second most common sexually trans-mitted disease.

 Tip: *It is very unlikely that the answer will be given away in the next question of the station.*

Bacterial vaginosis, the second most common answer, is the com-monest cause of vaginal discharge but not the commonest infection.

B➤ 1. False
2. True
3. True

1
1
1

A third of candidates have gained all three marks. Part 2 was the one answered incorrectly the most frequently. There is increasing evidence to show a higher rate of postoperative infection (endo-metritis, salpingitis) after suction termination if *Chlamydia* found on endocervical swab is not treated. A single dose of tetracycline is inadequate cover. Atopy enhances infection.

C➤ Any three of the following:

3

1. Pelvic inflammatory disease, leading to tubal damage
2. Chronic pelvic pain (CPP)
3. Ectopic pregnancy
4. Tubal infertility
5. Fitz-Hugh–Curtis syndrome (perihepatitis)

Again, well answered with just under half getting all the parts correct. If candidates listed dyspareunia we counted it as correct under the heading of chronic pelvic pain.

A small number offered neonatal chlamydial eye infection. This was not accepted because it is not a long-term complication of the host.

D➤ 1. Cervical wart viral infection, raised cauliflower lesions
2. Cervical dysplasia
   or
   Cervical carcinoma

1
1

Whilst we felt this to be a difficult photograph, over 65% of candi-dates were in fact correct. Most answered carcinoma of the cervix for the second half of this question.

 Howlers! Endometriosis; anal warts.

ANSWERS/COMMENTS

Score

E➤ Any one of the following:

1

1. Young age of first intercourse
2. Cigarette smoking
3. Multiple sexual partners
4. Immunosuppression

Out of the four possible predisposing factors, smoking was the answer most commonly given. Once a woman has been given the information that her smear shows cervical intraepithelial neoplasia (CIN), the question is often asked 'What is the cause of these abnormal cells?' The clinician must be ready with a factual answer that does not embarrass or distress her.

There are strong epidemiological associations between CIN and sexual behaviour. Women with this condition are more likely to have had early sexual experience, multiple sexual partners and sexually transmitted disease. The male partners of these women are likely to have had a similar sexual history. Epidemiological associations, however, never prove causation. Many women who develop CIN have only had one sexual partner.

Numerous epidemiological case-control population studies have shown an association between cigarette smoking and cervical cancer. The relative risk for developing this tumour in smokers, compared to non-smokers, has been calculated as fourfold after adjustment for risk factors. The risk remains elevated in ex-smokers.

There is uncertainty about the association between CIN and the different methods of contraception. Any epidemiological study must control for all the variables and accurately determine sexual histories for study and control cases. Available studies indicate that women on the combined oral contraceptive pill have a higher incidence of CIN than women using barrier methods. This may be partly explained, however, by the degree of exposure to seminal fluid. A male factor has long been sought as an aetiological component of the development of CIN. Recent work has looked at the possible role of immunosuppression by human seminal plasma in the aetiology of cervical neoplasia.

QUESTIONS

Study the accompanying menstrual calendar submitted by a 37-year-old lady who declares bitterly that her life has now become very difficult following her laparoscopic sterilization one year ago.

A► List the three features this chart demonstrates.

1.

2.

3.

B► List three possible causes for this lady's problems that could be diagnosed on a vaginal speculum examination.

1.

2.

3.

C► Given that the speculum examination was normal, how would you proceed now?

1. Perform a cervical smear.

   Yes/No

2. Refer for hysteroscopy.

   Yes/No

3. Perform a vaginal examination.

   Yes/No

4. Perform a pelvic ultrasound.

   Yes/No

QUESTIONS

Example

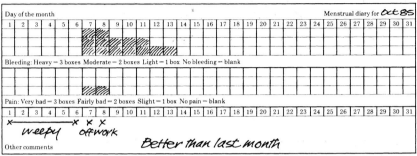

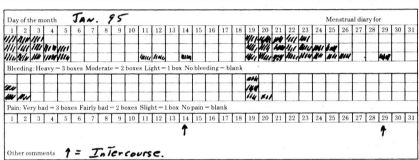

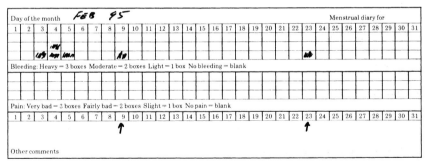

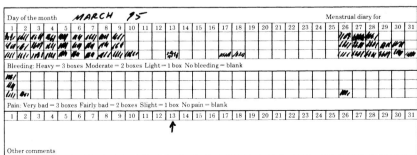

ANSWERS/COMMENTS

	Score

A➤ Any three of the following:

Score **3**

1. Intermenstrual bleeding
2. Postcoital bleeding
3. Dysfunctional uterine bleeding — heavy, irregular menses
4. Dysmenorrhoea

This question only requires you to be able to read a menstrual calendar, yet in validation only 65% of candidates scored three marks. Some candidates listed heavy bleeding and irregular bleeding as separate answers. They only scored two marks. This may seem harsh, but heavy irregular bleeding is the most obvious fact to elicit from a menstrual calendar. The authors wanted some evidence that more subtle symptoms would not be missed. A lot of information *can* be gleaned from charts like this if properly used.

 Tip: The examiners are instructed to give marks for the first three answers offered only. A number of candidates listed premenstrual tension, but this is only in the example at the top of the page and not in the months filled by the patient. You must study the charts carefully before starting to answer.

B➤ Any three of the following:

3

1. Cervical ectropion/cervicitis
2. Cervical polyp
3. Cervical carcinoma
4. Pedunculated fibroid

In validation over 60% of candidates gave correct answers.

ANSWERS/COMMENTS

C➤ 1. Yes   **1**
2. Yes   **1**
3. Yes   **1**
4. No   **1**

The guidelines for use of hysteroscopy suggest that this is not necessary for patients under 40 years of age. However, this refers to cases of heavy regular bleeding. It is appropriate to investigate the irregular loss of the patient in this case.

Some candidates offered ultrasound, presumably to exclude fibroids. An internal examination should be sufficient to exclude these.

QUESTIONS

A 21-year-old woman presents with an eight-month history of secondary amenorrhoea. She has had a milky discharge from her breasts for the past four months. General physical examination is unremarkable. Both breasts appear normal; milk can be expressed from the left breast. Pelvic examination is normal.

A➤ What is the likely diagnosis?

B➤ What additional specific physical finding would you look for on examination?

C➤ What key investigation would you perform?

D➤ What would be your first line of treatment?

E➤ List two other ways in which this condition might present.

1.

2.

F➤ Other causes of secondary amenorrhoea include:

1. hypothyroidism.

   True/False

2. Turner syndrome.

   True/False

3. Bulimia.

   True/False

4. Asherman syndrome.

   True/False

ANSWERS/COMMENTS

	Score

A➤ Hyperprolactinaemia

Score: **1**

In validation, many answered 'galactorrhoea'. This is a symptom or physical finding, not a diagnosis.

☞ *Tip: If the information is in the stem it is unlikely to be one of the answers.*

Howlers! Pregnancy, polycystic ovarian syndrome.

B➤ Visual field defects

Score: **1**

The specific defect is bitemporal hemianopia but a mark was given for visual field defect. A number of candidates have answered 'tunnel vision'. This is not correct.

C➤ Prolactin

Score: **1**

Again, basic information is required. Sadly, some candidates have tried to be too clever by asking for CAT and MRI scans. It is necessary to establish a diagnosis of hyperprolactinaemia before ordering these expensive diagnostic tests. The clue is in the words '**key** investigation'.

D➤ Bromocriptine

Score: **1**

In validation, this question was well answered, with 75% of candidates giving the correct answer.

Howlers! Duct dilation; combined oral contraceptive; clomid.

E➤ Any two of the following:

Score: **2**

1. Headaches
2. Visual disturbances
3. Infertility

Some candidates gave headache and visual disturbance as a single answer, scoring only one mark.

F➤
1. True — **1**
2. False — **1**
3. True — **1**
4. True — **1**

Turner syndrome is a cause of primary amenorrhoea.

QUESTIONS

A 34-year-old mother attends your surgery seven days after the delivery of her third child. The pregnancy and delivery were uncomplicated. She has no relevant past medical history and takes no regular medications.

A► If she is not breast feeding and wishes to start the combined oral contraceptive pill, which of the following would you suggest to maximize its efficacy?

1. Start it at once (a week following delivery).

   Yes/No

2. Start it following her six-week postnatal visit.

   Yes/No

3. Start it on the first day of her first period.

   Yes/No

4. Start it on the fifth day of her first period.

   Yes/No

5. Start it three weeks after delivery.

   Yes/No

B► In a breastfeeding mother with well-established lactation, would you recommend the following methods of contraception?

1. Depoprogesterone injection.

   Yes/No

2. Norplant.

   Yes/No

3. Levonorgestrel-containing IUCD.

   Yes/No

QUESTIONS

C➤ If she wishes to use natural methods of contraception and is breast feeding:

1. Should she consider herself infertile until her first menstruation?

   Yes/No

2. If she supplements the night feed, will this have an effect on her fertility?

   Yes/No

ANSWERS/COMMENTS

Score

A➤ 1. No   1
     2. No   1
     3. No   1
     4. No   1
     5. Yes   1

The optimal time for a mother who is not breast feeding to start the oral contraceptive pill is three weeks after delivery. Two percent of mothers who do not breast feed will ovulate before 28 days and 33% will ovulate before their first period. In one study the mean duration of amenorrhoea was 59 days. Oestrogen levels remain elevated for 5–7 days following delivery, therefore starting the pill before three weeks will increase the risk of thromboembolism.

B➤ 1. Yes   1
     2. Yes   1
     3. Yes   1

All progesterone-containing products can be used by breastfeeding mothers.

C➤ 1. No   1
     2. Yes. Once supplementary feeds are introduced, 50% ovulate within the next 16 weeks even though lactation is maintained.   1

This question has been well answered. Ovulation does not occur provided full lactation is maintained. It appears that six or more episodes of sucking in 24 hours and a reduced interval between feeds are the important factors in delaying ovulation. Once supplementary feeds are introduced half will ovulate within three months even though lactation is maintained.

QUESTIONS

A 62-year-old patient attends your surgery complaining of a watery bloodstained discharge for the first time since her menopause which was at the age of 50. She has had no previous gynaecological problems.

A➤ List four questions you would wish to ask her to further differentiate the problem.

1. _____

2. _____

3. _____

4. _____

B➤ What is the most common cause of postmenopausal bleeding?

_____

C➤ List three investigations that could be carried out to aid your diagnosis.

1. _____

2. _____

3. _____

D➤ Assuming that the answer for B was the correct diagnosis:

1. How would you treat this condition?

_____

2. What common problem can further complicate this condition?

_____

ANSWERS/COMMENTS

Score
4

A➤ Any four of the following:

1. Is she taking HRT?
2. Is there a history of carcinoma of the breast resulting in tamoxifen therapy?
3. Has she had recent intercourse?
4. When was her last smear test and what was the result?
5. Is she sure the discharge is vaginal?
6. Does she have a ring pessary in situ?

This question has been very poorly answered. You are expected to ask questions that would help you arrive at a possible cause of the bleeding.

 Howlers! Age of menarche; does she snore?

 Tip: Read the question. Candidates offered: is it a postmenopausal bleed? any previous episodes? is it intermittent? These are in the stem.

 Differentiator: Many candidates have suggested: smelly discharge; does it itch? presence of pain. These do not really help to differentiate the problem. These can all be associated with both endometrial and cervical carcinoma. A history of recent intercourse should be included as watery, bloodstained discharge may be due to haematospermia (also contact bleeding from a cervical carcinoma).

B➤ Atrophic vaginitis

1

Only 50% of candidates have given atrophic vaginitis. Endometrial carcinoma is the major concern but it is not the most common cause of postmenopausal bleeding.

C➤ Any three of the following:

3

1. Smear if no recent result is available
2. Vaginal probe ultrasound, for endometrial thickness
3. Endometrial sampling
4. Hysteroscopy

There are several possible causes of the lady's watery, bloodstained discharge but candidates only listed tests that would exclude endometrial carcinoma.

ANSWERS/COMMENTS

Score

 *Tip: Pipelle and D&C both provide the same information. In this type of question you will usually be expected to give three different **types** of tests. Hysteroscopy does allow visualization and the authors have generously allowed this as a separate answer. In reality, hysteroscopy is unlikely to be performed without endometrial sampling.*

Several studies have evaluated the most efficient methods of investigating postmenopausal bleeding. Some centres have set up a specific postmenopausal bleeding clinic, providing a 'one-stop' service, based on ultrasonography and endometrial biopsy with a management protocol. Others have established an outpatient endoscopy service to complement formal endometrial biopsy.

Vaginal probe ultrasound enhances resolution if the patient can tolerate this approach. The normal postmenopausal uterus contains no tissue, therefore there should be a clear difference between this and a uterine cavity containing endometrial pathology. In most studies all abnormal endometrial change has occurred above an endometrial thickness of 5 mm. One study estimated a positive predictive value of 87% and a sensitivity of 100% using this cut-off measurement.

Outpatient endometrial sampling may be by means of Vabra aspiration using a suction curette or by Gynaecheck or Pipelle device; all these techniques are fairly well tolerated. The curette is narrow and there is no need for cervical dilation. A pain similar to dysmenorrhoea is often experienced. Several studies have compared one form of endometrial sampling with another and found little difference in tumour detection rates.

Endometrial biopsy techniques are easily learned and are safe. Formal examination under anaesthesia and D&C should be performed if bleeding recurs after an outpatient endometrial biopsy has failed to demonstrate an abnormality.

D➤ 1. Prescribe a course of topical oestrogens.
   2. Secondary bacterial vaginosis. Treat this with the appropriate antibiotic.

1
1

This question has been poorly answered because candidates invariably gave the wrong answer to B.

QUESTIONS

Weekly Progress Chart

Name ___MRS BLACK___ Week beginning ___1/3/96___

KEY ▢ _____ ▢ _____

SPECIAL INSTRUCTIONS *Purchase a cheap plastic measuring jug – measure urine output (in mls) on 3 separate days. Choose days that are convenient to you. They do not have to be next to each other. Fill in the volume voided against the time, for a full 24 hours. Give an estimate of volume drunk each day.*

Time	SUNDAY	MONDAY	TUESDAY	WEDNESDAY	THURSDAY	FRIDAY	SATURDAY
6am				150	6.30 100		
7am	150	120	7.30	110			130
8am							8.30 90
9am	50			90			
10am	25		10.30	100	w		120
11am							
Noon	70			150			200
1pm			1.30	w 100	(shopping)		1.30 90 (going out)
2pm	150		2.15	60			2.40 70 (Tescos)
3pm (2.45)	70						ww
4pm		w		150			150 (waiting for bus)
5pm	150						5.30 80
6pm (6.30)	90			120	w		
7pm		w			(asleep)		100
8pm			8.30	100			7.30 30 (going out)
9pm	200	(watching TV)					150
10pm (10.30)	108			130			60
11pm							10.50 50
Midnight	150			75			200
1am							
2am	200						150 w
3am (3.30)	175 w (asleep)	w (asleep)		200 (asleep)			
4am							
5am	150			120			120
TOTAL FLUID INTAKE		7 mugs		4 cups 5 mugs			2 lagers 4 cups 2 mugs

Mark w for wet.   ww if a real gush occurred

QUESTIONS

Mrs Black attended your surgery a month ago complaining of urinary leakage. You found her a rather vague historian and as time was short, sent her away to complete a filling/voiding chart. She now returns and presents her voiding chart for you to examine.

Study the attached chart and answer the following questions.

A➤ From the information you have in front of you, what do you consider to be the likely diagnosis?

B➤ Given that Mrs Black does leak, outline three questions that you would need to ask to estimate the severity of the problem.

  1. _____

  2. _____

  3. _____

C➤ What two tests would you order to help make a diagnosis?

  1. _____

  2. _____

D➤ Outline two treatment strategies for the management of this condition.

  1. _____

  2. _____

E➤ Name two health care professionals that you may wish to involve in this case.

  1. _____

  2. _____

ANSWERS/COMMENTS

| | Score |

A► **Detrusor instability (unstable bladder; urge incontinence)**   Score: **1**

A third of candidates have answered 'stress incontinence'. The voiding chart shows frequent voids with small volumes passed. It is true that some ladies with bladder neck weakness compensate by voiding frequently, to minimize the leakage when it occurs, but this is 'reading things in'.

 Tip: Take the medical evidence at face value!

One candidate has answered 'retention with overflow'. This is a possibility but not the most likely diagnosis in a woman.

B► **Any three of the following:**   **3**

1. How socially incapacitating is the problem (e.g. does the patient have to avoid certain activities such as dancing, exercise? Does she have to limit the length of time she is out of the house, etc.?)?
2. How severe is the leakage (e.g. does it amount to a few drops? Does it wet her underwear? Does it gush, i.e. run down her legs?)?
3. Does she wear pads for protection (if yes, how many)?
4. Frequency of the loss (per day; 2–3 times per week)?

Fifty percent of candidates have managed to get two out of three correct. Those who asked if she leaked with coughing and sneezing missed the point of the question.

 Tip: You are asked to assess the severity of the urinary leakage, not the cause of it.

C► 1. Midstream urine for culture   **1**
2. Videocystometry – filling/voiding cystometry   **1**

A minority offered pad testing. This would serve to further quantify the loss but would not provide a diagnosis.

 Howler! Micturating cystogram.

ANSWERS/COMMENTS

D➤ Any two of the following:

1. Anticholinergics
2. Bladder retraining/biofeedback
3. Unomax stimulator
4. Psychotherapy/hypnotherapy
5. Physiotherapy

Obviously, those who felt the problem was stress incontinence did not do well in this question. The mainstay of treatment for detrusor instability is anticholinergic therapy. Nevertheless, medication can cause significant side effects: dry mouth, diplopia, constipation and oesophageal dysmotility. Some women cannot tolerate a sufficient dose to provide symptom relief.

Behavioural therapy for instability is based on the premise that loss of bladder control is the result of maladaptive learnt behaviour. Cortical bladder control has been lost or never established. Bladder drill is the most commonly used form and can be very effective. However, co-operation and motivation are mandatory. The symptoms are controlled by forcing the patient to regain control of her bladder by a rigid timed voiding schedule in which the time between voids is gradually increased.

A number of studies have demonstrated the effectiveness of acupuncture in the management of nocturnal enuresis. More recently, it has been shown to achieve symptomatic cure in over 70% of patients with idiopathic detrusor instability and predominantly daytime symptoms. Electrical stimulation has also been shown to improve detrusor instability. Surgery should always be the last resort, usually clam ileocystoplasty, which will necessitate intermittent self-catheterization postoperatively.

E➤ 1. Continence advisors
2. Physiotherapists

1
1

It is important that GPs know what professional help is available for women with urinary problems. There is evidence to show that physiotherapy can be helpful in the management of instability, by overriding the urge. A senior physiotherapist will thoroughly assess the patient and plan a full treatment programme. Continence advisors will teach bladder control programmes and biofeedback techniques.

REST STATION

INTERACTIVE STATION

Instructions to candidate

You have known Mrs Thomas, who runs the village post office, for some years. She is 65 years old, a rather shy, demure and quietly spoken woman.

She has made an appointment to see you today following her recent consultation with the consultant gynaecologist at the district general hospital in the nearby market town.

You have received a letter from him outlining his plans to perform a radical vulvectomy.

A copy of the histology report from her original biopsy has already been sent to you (see attached).

Please answer Mrs Thomas's questions.

GYNAECOLOGICAL HISTOPATHOLOGY CYTOLOGY REQUEST/REPORT

Consultant	Ward/Dept.	
Bloggs	CURIE	Mrs Thomas Age 65

Clinical condition (please tick)					Date of previous smear 11/93				Clinical information (please tick)		Cervix	
Oral contraceptive	Current	Past	Never		Neg. ✓	Susp.	Malig.		L.M.P.	Discharge	Normal	
Other hormones	Specify									Haemorrhage	Eroded	
I.U.C.D.					No. of live births				Cycle	Post-coital	Cervicitis	
Routine smear					No. of still births (excluding abortions)		3		Menopausal ✓	Post-menopausal	Polyps	
Gynae symptoms										Inter-menstrual	Malignant	
Pregnant	Nature of specimen Vulval biopsy								Collected at			
Post-natal (under 12 weeks)	Symptoms and clinical diagnosis-								on			
Previous R.T.	Pruritus vulvae											

Peri-clitoral lesion biopsy

FOR LAB USE ONLY	Report
Lab. No	
Received :	Macro – 3cm x 2cm Ulcerating lesion
Date	
Time	Micro – Moderately differentiated squamous cell carcinoma
Trimmed :	Invading to 15 mm
Tissues processed :	Some perivascular infiltration

RO77-70

Date 10/6/95		Signature

Date of request 6/6/95	Signature of Dr. making request	GYNAECOLOGY HISTOPATHOLOGY CYTOLOGY

INTERACTIVE STATION

Instructions to actress

You are Mrs Thomas, a naturally shy and rather timid 65-year-old lady. You have come to talk to your general practitioner following a recent consultation at the local hospital. You found the examination by a male gynaecologist very embarrassing. When he told you that you had vulval cancer your mind went blank and you cannot remember any of the ensuing conversation. When you got home you wrote down a list of questions that you would like your family doctor to answer.

You will conduct the interview with your doctor in a careful and methodical fashion. Though you are shy, you do want to know precisely where you will stand after surgery.

You will be quite persistent, should the doctor show any signs of reluctance in answering your questions, although the discussion regarding sexual function will cause you some embarrassment.

Your questions are as follows (all need to be covered):

1. Please explain to me what the operation entails.
2. How disfiguring will this procedure be?
3. How long am I likely to remain in hospital?
4. What will sexual relations with my husband be like afterwards? Will we still enjoy a good sex life?

Instructions to examiner

This station is designed to test the candidate's ability to conduct an interview with sensitivity and compassion, whilst still providing accurate and detailed medical information.

The examiner will have copies of the instructions to both actress and candidate.

ANSWERS/COMMENTS

	Score

Marks awarded by the actress

A➤ Empathy/compassion 0/1/2

0	1	2
None		Good

B➤ Ability to explain treatment in lay terms 0/1/2

0	1	2
Poorly understandable		Easily understandable

C➤ Felt confidence in candidate/would like to see again 0/1/2

0	1	2
Poor		Excellent

Marks awarded by the examiner

1. The operation entails removal of labia/removal of clitoral hood and clitoris/bilateral groin dissection en bloc for inguinal nodes. The size and site of the lesion may dictate whether the low portion of the urethra, vagina or external anal sphincters are resected. — **1**
2. The degree of disfigurement depends on the extent of surgery (see above). — **1**
3. Length of hospital stay 18–21 days. — **1**
4. Sexual function is preserved to some extent. If the vaginal tissues are kept stretched, there would be adequate vaginal capacity. Clitoral stimulation is not possible, but cervical stimulation can still occur. — **1**

This is one of the stations in our series that has been piloted on three occasions. Quite a considerable quantity of medical information has to be demonstrated during the interview and candidates have commented that it is difficult to get through all the information required and demonstrate interactive communication skills in the time allowed. We have therefore redesigned the marking system to aid the examiner and latterly to allow the actress to be involved in scoring too. For this station the actresses have been medical students or volunteered SHO!

The candidates have certainly performed differently during the last three validation processes. On the first occasion there was almost universal walkout from this station. Candidates either burst out laughing and said they knew nothing about the topic whatsoever or looked aghast and with a shamed face said that they would have to either send the patient back to the hospital for the consultant to see again or consult another colleague in

ANSWERS/COMMENTS

the practice. Many apologized and said that there was little point continuing with the station since it was merely wasting the actress's time.

The discrepancy in performance is probably related to the change in scoring systems. Six points can now be scored on the interactive skills. There is a maximum of only four points now available for accuracy of medical facts. Lack of medical knowledge, however, was often reflected in the score from the actress. She was able to sense when a candidate had no idea about this topic and therefore did not score highly when asked if she felt confident with the doctor or if she wished to see this doctor again.

Candidates have complained that this seems to be a difficult station. The counterargument must be made that a certain basic level of knowledge must be obtained to enable general practitioners to counsel patients who are obviously agitated and distressed, having received the diagnosis of cancer, and who turn to the doctor whom they know best for support. This scenario could well form the basis of a structured oral, when all the marks would be awarded for factual information.

QUESTIONS

William is three days old and you are asked by the midwife to visit. Mother is very concerned that he has been jaundiced for 24 hours. He was born by normal vaginal delivery in the local maternity unit and was discharged within 36 hours quite well.

A➤ 1. What is the most likely cause of the jaundice?

2. What are the physiological/pathological reasons underlying it?

B➤ 1. If the jaundice had started on day 5 when the child became unwell, what would be the most likely aetiology?

2. List four investigations which would be essential.

  a

  b

  c

  d

C➤ List three common causes of prolonged jaundice after ten days.

  1.

  2.

  3.

ANSWERS/COMMENTS

		Score
A➤	1. Physiological jaundice	1
	2. One of the following:	1

   a Glucuronyl transferase inhibition preventing conjugation

   b High initial Hb at delivery which is falling

Everyone seemed aware that physiological causes were the most likely reasons for jaundice at this stage and had a good understanding of the mechanisms involved. This would be regarded as a 'standard stem', i.e. one that allowed every candidate to make a few marks.

		Score
B➤	1. Sepsis	1
	2. a Liver function tests including split bilirubin	1
	b Full blood count	1
	c Blood cultures	1
	d Suprapubic aspiration	1

All candidates identified sepsis as the most likely cause of jaundice on day 5 but had differing views on the four *essential* investigations. Blood cultures and liver function tests were remembered by most (not everyone specified split bilirubin).

The need to exclude urine infection was generally recognized, but most candidates were overoptimistic in the co-operation they anticipated from a three-day-old infant.

 Howler! *Requesting a midstream urine! A suprapubic aspirate (SPA) is, of course, more realistic.*

Several candidates offered thyroid function test. Hypothyroidism can produce jaundice but is not the *most likely* cause on day 5.

ANSWERS/COMMENTS

	Score

C➤ 1. Breast milk jaundice — **1**
2. Dehydration — **1**
3. ABO incompatibility — **1**

Pitfall: *When asked to produce three **common** causes of prolonged jaundice, glucose-6-phosphatase dehydrogenase deficiency (G6PD deficiency) is not perhaps the most sensible choice to offer. Read the stem carefully. Similarly, congenital biliary atresia is correct but relatively rare.*

Just over half the candidates included breast milk jaundice, approximately 25% covered ABO incompatibility and only one candidate mentioned dehydration.

Sepsis in various forms (urinary tract infections, hepatitis, etc.) was the most common answer, despite the fact that it had been the answer to the previous question.

Tip: *It is unlikely the examiners will expect the same answer twice.*

It is worth mentioning that this station has been piloted three times: twice with DRCOG trainees and once with the entire paediatric department at one of the authors' hospitals.

INTERACTIVE STATION

Instructions to actress

You are a 35-year-old Italian with two children and are rather highly strung. You work hard helping in your husband's restaurant. A recent smear performed in your GP's surgery suggested CIN3. You were advised on referral for colposcopy. This was performed last week at the local hospital and biopsies were taken. You have an appointment to return to the hospital next week but you cannot wait. You are absolutely convinced that you have cancer (and will pursue this line of discussion) and that there is a conspiracy to hide this from you. You are tearful and you have no-one else to turn to – your husband is too busy with his restaurant. You find it hard to listen to the doctor and take in what you are told. You need a lot of persuading to calm down.

Instructions to candidate

You have known Rosita, aged 35 years, since she was a child. She is now happily married with two children and helps run her husband's success-ful restaurant just down the road from your surgery. A recent smear test performed by your practice nurse suggested CIN3 and Rosita has under-gone urgent colposcopy. She has now made an urgent appointment to see you and the reception staff have warned you that she is very distressed. You have talked to the senior registrar this morning and know she has CIN3 confirmed on both colposcopic biopsies and colposcopy assess-ment. You must attempt to calm her down and explain the meaning of the term CIN3, how it differs from cancer and how likely CIN3 is, or is not, to become cancer.

Instructions to examiner

You have been issued with a score sheet testing the candidate's commu-nication skills. You must also confer with the actress afterwards with regard to the candidate's ability to conduct the interview. You will assess the candidate's understanding of CIN3 and ability to explain dyskaryosis to the patient and to reassure the patient. Accuracy of medical knowledge and ability to calm a near-hysterical patient are being tested simultane-ously here.

ANSWERS/COMMENTS

Marks awarded by the examiner

A► Listening skills

0	1	2
Did not listen		Did listen, did not interrupt and good use of silence

B► Empathy

0	1	2
Did not acknowledge patient's distress		Did acknowledge distress with an empathetic manner

C► Exploring the patient's understanding

0	1	2
Doctor fails to explore what patient understands of situation		Doctor fully explores patient's understanding

D► Support

0	1	2
Doctor offered no/little support		Support offered or reassurance given. Practice nurse offered as back-up. Offer of visit at home later

E► Understanding of presenting pathology demonstrated and clearly explained to patient in understandable terminology

0	1	2
No idea		Good grasp of term CIN3

Explanation should include:

- Discussion of the meaning of the term CIN3. This is a histological definition of severe dysplasia. (Dyskaryosis is a cytological term.)
- The basement membrane is intact. This is not invasive cancer.
- Studies have shown that less than 40% of patients with CIN3 develop cancer after 20 years.
- The evidence from the hospital should be stressed – smear, biopsy and colposcopic appearance all agree. More sinister pathology is unlikely to be missed.

ANSWERS/COMMENTS

- Describe the histological appearance and how it differs from cancer.
- Describe the colposcopic appearance and staining techniques.

This is a common problem that is often encountered in general practice. Patients often assume the worst and will interpret even a cytology report showing CIN1 as meaning something very sinister.

Generally, candidates have shown a good degree of empathy and understanding. Listening skills, however, have not been particularly well demonstrated and the explanations given varied considerably in their accuracy. A number of candidates have given the impression that CIN3 can develop into cancer very quickly and some have had a very poor understanding of what dyskaryosis means.

Dyskaryosis is a cytological diagnosis which refers to individual cells' appearance. The critieria judged are enlargement and hyperchromasia of the nuclei, with uneven chromatin distribution, irregular nuclear membrane and multinucleation.

Dysplasia is a histological diagnosis which describes abnormalities of the epithelium. Part of the thickness of the epithelium has been replaced by cells showing varying degrees of atypia. In CIN1 (mild dysplasia), for example, the upper two thirds of the epithelium exhibit relatively good differentiation. There are mild nuclear abnormalities, most marked in the basal layer. There are a few mitotic figures, confined to the basal third. CIN3, by contrast, exhibits nuclear abnormalities throughout the full thickness of the epithelium. Mitotic figures may be numerous and at all levels. Maturation is confined to the superficial one third of the epithelium or is absent. The basement membrane is, however, intact.

Obviously, a full-thickness biopsy provides more accurate and detailed information than cytology. There is a wide variation but there is at least a 5–10% false-negative smear rate. This may be due to an error in taking the smear, poor sampling or fixing techniques or an error in interpretation by the cytologist. Finally, the size of the lesion may be too small so that very few cells are exfoliated.

False-positive smears may be due to laboratory error, but a positive smear with negative colposcopy may represent undetected lesions not seen at colposcopy, as they are higher within the endocervical canal. If a smear is positive but colposcopic assessment is negative, the smear should be repeated. If the same abnormality is detected, a cone biopsy is indicated.

ANSWERS/COMMENTS

Colposcopy allows detailed examination of the cervix to take place under magnification. Using examination under white light and green filter, to facilitate identifying vessel patterns and utilizing different staining techniques to highlight abnormal areas, accurate colposcopically directed biopsies can be taken. The squamocolumnar junction can be identified and the size and depth of an area of abnormality assessed.

Treatment can then be planned and often initiated, as well as diagnosis enhanced.

Circuit E

QUESTIONS

Score

A► Name two different methods for providing contraceptive cover for three months at a time.

1. _____

2. _____

B► List three ways in which the newer of these two alternatives offers advantages over the older method.

1. _____

2. _____

3. _____

C► Name two different types of contraception offering contraceptive cover for five years at a time.

1. _____

2. _____

D► Which of these would be:

1. most suitable for a patient with a history of pelvic inflammatory disease?

_____

2. unsuitable for a patient with a large fibroid uterus?

_____

E► Which of these methods requires the practitioner to have a certificate of competence and a minimum rate of 50 fittings per year to practise?

_____

ANSWERS/COMMENTS

Score

A➤ 1. Depo-Provera (depot medroxyprogesterone acetate)   **1**
2. The Fem-ring   **1**

 Differentiator: *It is accepted that the Fem-ring is still in the development stage but candidates would be expected to have heard of it.*

This has not been well answered; less than 5% of candidates gave Fem-ring. There has been a great deal of interest in the contraceptive vaginal ring. The progestogerone-only ring looks similar to a vaginal ring pessary and is 5–6 cm in diameter. Several progestogens have been tried. Fem-ring releases 20 mg of levonorgestrel locally each day. It is absorbed through the vaginal mucosa, avoiding the peak dose to the liver given by oral preparations and the associated fluctuating blood levels. The ring is effective for three months' use. The main contraceptive activity is to thicken the cervical mucus. There is a failure rate of 3–4 per 100 woman-years. Multicentre studies have demonstrated a 7% expulsion rate, mainly related to pelvic wall laxity. Continuation rates are between 50% and 75%; irregular bleeding has been the problem quoted most often. Some centres have noted asymptomatic erythematous vaginal wall patches in some users. This could be due to pressure effects or local progestogen effects and investigations are currently being undertaken.

A number of candidates offered the combined pill. This will provide contraception for three months, as indeed will any method if used correctly. The question specifically asks for methods that provide cover for three months at a time. Later in the station, you are asked for types of contraceptives providing five-year cover. This should alert you to the fact that the examiner is looking for specific methods.

B➤ 1. Reversibility   **1**
2. Much less risk of amenorrhoea/no concern regarding osteoporosis   **1**
3. No problems with delay in return to fertility   **1**

As A has been so poorly answered, few have done well in this section.

ANSWERS/COMMENTS

Score

C➤ 1. Some of the coils, i.e.:   1
   a Levonova
   b Nova-T/Novaguard
   c Multi-load Cu 375
   d Mirena

   2. Norplant (levonorgestrel, 38 mg per capsule)   1

Most candidates have suggested coils; many have offered Norplant
(more than 60%).

Norplant is a low-dose, reversible, progestogen-only implant that
lasts five years. It has been available in the United Kingdom since
1993. There are more than one million users in the United States of
America and more than four million users worldwide.

Norplant consists of six small, flexible, sealed capsules which are
placed, in a fan-shaped pattern, in the subdermal layer of the upper
inner aspect of the woman's non-dominant arm, approximately 8 cm
from the medial epicondyle. No stitches are necessary in the wounds
made for Norplant insertion/removal.

Each capsule contains 38 mg of levonorgestrel. Initially, 85 µg of
levonorgestrel is released daily, falling to 50 µg by six months and
35 µg by 18 months. Norplant has three main methods by which it
provides contraception: thickening of cervical mucus, suppression of
ovulation in 50% of cycles (particularly in the first year of usage) and,
in those cycles where ovulation does occur, there appears to be
endometrial luteal phase deficiency, inhibiting implantation.

Norplant has a low pregnancy rate, 0.2 per 100 continuing users for
the first year, with a cumulative pregnancy rate of 3.9 per 100 users
over five years.

Once Norplant is removed, the contraceptive effect ceases almost
immediately. It appears to be an acceptable method of contraception
if women are counselled adequately first.

The majority of women (60–80%) will experience some change in
bleeding pattern during the first year. This may be prolonged bleeding, spotting or amenorrhoea. The menstrual irregularities tend to
settle with time. Occasionally, women complain of headache, mastalgia, dizziness or hair growth (5–10%).

Capsule expulsion and infection at the implant site are uncommon.
Much publicity has been given to a few cases where retrieval of the

ANSWERS/COMMENTS

Score

capsules proved difficult. Often the capsules were inserted too deeply or removal was attempted by inexperienced health professionals. This method of contraception only works well and is acceptable if insertion and removal are performed by fully trained clinicians.

Ideally, Norplant should be inserted on the first day of a period or within five days of a miscarriage. If it is inserted at any other time additional contraceptive cover is required for seven days.

In the future new implants may become available, offering contraceptive cover for 2–3 years. Two possible contenders will be biodegradable, preventing the need for removal.

 Howlers! Diaphragm; condoms.

D► 1. Norplant   1
    2. The coil   1

E► The coil   1

QUESTIONS

You are called to see a primagravida of 30 weeks' gestation who has arrived on the labour ward contracting moderately every 4–5 minutes. The patient has always been regarded as being rather small for dates.

A➤ Management issues.

1. Would you give ritodrine if the patient was on methyldopa for pre-eclampsia?

   Yes/No

2. Maternal thyrotoxicosis would not be a contraindication to the use of a tocolytic.

   Yes/No

3. Right-sided heart failure may occur if ritodrine is given to the mother after betamethasone has been administered to aid maturation of the foetal lungs.

   Yes/No

B➤ What particular factor in this case would make you rather wary of halting labour?

C➤ Assuming that the membranes were ruptured, the cervix was 2 cm dilated and there was no maternal pyrexia:

1. under what circumstances would you give a tocolytic?

2. Why?

D➤ What percentage of normal vaginal deliveries result from preterm labour?

%

QUESTIONS

Score

E➤ What percentage of neonatal deaths are a result of:

1. prematurity?

_____ %

2. congenital abnormalities?

_____ %

3. hypoxia?

_____ %

ANSWERS/COMMENTS

	Score

A➤ 1. No — 1

2. No — 1

3. Yes — 1

During validation, some candidates felt the question was too clinical; nevertheless, it was quite well answered. The question relates to labour management you should have observed during your time as an SHO and is regarded as fair. There are always a number of approaches to any clinical problem. However, if a mother presented in preterm labour with a small baby and pre-eclampsia most obstetricians would not attempt to halt the labour. Watch the double negative in question A.2. The absolute contraindications to tocolysis are thyroid disease, cardiac disease, severe hypertension, sickle cell disease and chorioamnionitis. Right-sided heart failure is a well-documented complication of tocolytic use. Fluid balance must be carefully monitored and early signs of fluid overload acted upon.

B➤ The baby has been noted to be small for dates. It would be inappropriate to halt labour if there was a degree of placental insufficiency. — 1

Candidates have given a long list of general worrying factors. The question specifically asks about *this case*.

C➤ 1. There were inadequate neonatal care facilities on the site to cope with a 30-week foetus. — 1

2. To delay the labour long enough to effect an in utero transfer to another unit. — 1

Most candidates knew what was being asked of them. Tocolytics are justified to allow in utero transfer and to delay labour long enough to allow time for steroids to aid lung maturity.

 Howler! *Herpes simplex.*

D➤ 1. 5–10% — 1

E➤ 1. 60–70% — 1

2. 25–35% — 1

3. 5–10% — 1

Most candidates have just guessed these answers!

QUESTIONS

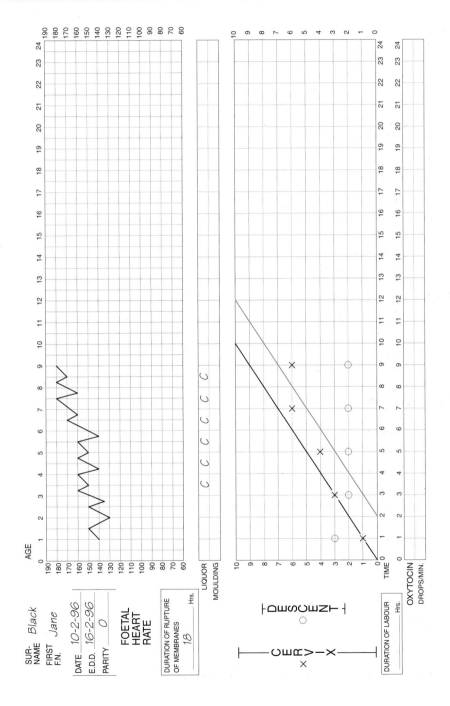

AGE

SUR-NAME _Black_
FIRST F.N. _Jane_

DATE _10-2-96_
E.D.D. _16-2-96_
PARITY _0_

FOETAL HEART RATE

DURATION OF RUPTURE OF MEMBRANES _18_ Hrs.

LIQUOR

MOULDING

DESCENT

DURATION OF LABOUR _____ Hrs.

OXYTOCIN

DROPS/MIN.

QUESTIONS

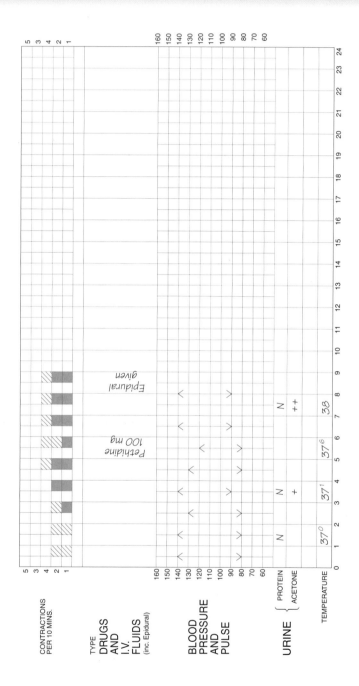

QUESTIONS

A➤ List the three main adverse features this partogram shows.

1. _____

2. _____

3. _____

B➤ In not more than two sentences, explain the most likely sequence of events that has led to the present foetal situation.

_____

_____

_____

C➤ What two essential steps would you take?

1. _____

2. _____

D➤ How would you correct this lady's ketoacidosis?

_____

_____

E➤ When would you reassess this mother (i.e. do the next vaginal examination)?

_____

_____

F➤ Define moulding.

_____

_____

ANSWERS/COMMENTS

	Score
A► 1. Foetal tachycardia	1
2. Failure to progress	1
3. Maternal pyrexia	1

 Tip: If asked for three features, you should try and list three **separate** *features, even if the question does not specifically say so. In this question, failure to progress, secondary arrest and poor uterine activity are all just a single feature and as such will only score one mark!*

B► Prolonged rupture of membranes. Early chorioamnionitis   **2**

Many candidates discussed aspects of failure to progress. This would not be accepted because failure to progress does not relate to the present foetal situation. The partogram contains the information that the membranes have been ruptured for 18 hours.

C► Any two of the following: **2**

1. Start syntocinon.
2. Reduce maternal pyrexia.
3. Commence antibiotics.

Most have mentioned augmentation; few have addressed the maternal pyrexia.

 Howlers! Rupture the membranes; forceps delivery; give analgesia.

The partogram already gives the information that the cervix is 6 cm dilated, that the membranes are ruptured and that the mother has an epidural. Read all the information you are given.

D► By giving a litre of 5% dextrose   **1**

Many candidates have suggested putting up a drip. A more specific answer is required.

E► Two hours after starting syntocinon   **1**

F► The degree to which the foetal skull bones are overlapped   **1**

The word 'overlap' must appear if the answer is to gain a mark. Many candidates talked about reshaping of the head or pressure on the head. These answers are too vague.

QUESTIONS

Jane is a 24-year-old girl who has attended your practice for ten years. She has a thick file because she is a bad asthmatic. Currently she takes beclomethasone diproprionate 50 µg, two puffs four times a day; salbutamol, two puffs four times a day and prednisolone, 5 mg a day. She is a non-smoker. She is keen to start a family and comes to discuss this with you.

A➤ What advice would you give Jane about the effects of pregnancy on her asthma?

_____

_____

_____

B➤ Jane asks if her asthma will affect the development of her baby.

Yes/No _____

C➤ Outline three steps you would take to achieve optimal control of her asthma before she becomes pregnant.

1. _____

2. _____

3. _____

D➤ Since she is very worried about labour, is she at an increased risk of having an acute asthma attack during her labour?

Yes/No _____

E➤ In this case, what are the special precautions that should be taken during labour?

_____

_____

QUESTIONS

Score

F▶ 1. Jane asks 'Is it better to breast feed rather than bottle feed my baby?'

   Yes/No

2. Is it safe to breast feed her baby while taking the medication listed above?

   Yes/No

G▶ Jane's partner is not asthmatic. What is the risk of her baby being affected with asthma in childhood?

%

ANSWERS/COMMENTS

Score

A▶ Pregnancy has no specific effect on asthma.   1

B▶ No   1

A and B have been answered very well.

Asthma is a very variable condition. Its severity depends on the patient's exposure to allergens and the presence of respiratory infections, both also dependent on the season of the year. In addition, the patient's emotional state is important. If sufficient patients are studied to allow for these other influences, pregnancy has no consistent effect on asthma. A number of studies have looked at the risk incurred by the foetus of asthmatic mothers. Some studies show a slight increase in prematurity in pregnancies of patients receiving corticosteroids. Others have mentioned a tendency to growth retardation, particularly amongst foetuses of mothers taking oral steroid therapy. These patients were more severely affected by asthma and may have been intermittently hypoxic. If there is an increased risk at all it is small and should not be exaggerated when counselling the individual patient.

 Tip: As the question has asked for a categorical 'yes' or 'no' answer as to whether asthma will affect the development of her baby, the answer must be 'no'. If the question had asked 'May there be an increased risk?' the answer would be 'yes'.

C▶ Any three of the following: 3

1. Increase dose of inhaled steroids
2. Try to wean off oral steroids
3. Regular peak flow readings
4. Refer to chest physician.

Most candidates have only managed to score one out of three.

 *Howlers! 'Avoid cigarettes' – the stem states she does not smoke. 'Treat infection' – what infection? Answers should refer to this specific case – '. . . to achieve optimal control of **her** asthma . . .'.*

D▶ No   1

ANSWERS/COMMENTS

	Score

E▶ Reasonable to give epidural to reduce the risk of general anaesthesia — **1**
or
Hydrocortisone cover, if on continuous steroid therapy for more than two weeks in the previous year

F▶ 1. Yes. Reduces risk of atopy — **1**
2. Yes — **1**

D, E and F have been well answered.

It is unusual for labour to be complicated by attacks of asthma. Possibly this is due to increased glucocorticoid and catecholamine output. Prostaglandin secretion during labour may also cause bronchodilation.

G▶ 5% — **1**

Generally, far too high a risk has been offered. Some candidates have said 50% and many 5–10%.

QUESTIONS

Score

Rose, who is 52 years old, attends your surgery for advice about hormone replacement therapy. She has quite severe menopausal symptoms, particularly vaginal dryness and dyspareunia. Her last period was three months ago. In the past she has had four children and suffered a deep venous thrombosis during the second pregnancy, which was never confirmed. There is no other relevant past medical or family history.

A➤ List three common routes of administering hormone replacement therapy.

1. _____

2. _____

3. _____

B➤ 1. Which first-line therapy would you use in this woman's case?

_____

2. State in not more than one sentence why you would choose this route.

_____

C➤ If this woman had presented with a history of recurrent idiopathic episodes of thrombosis, list four investigations you should perform before starting her on hormone replacement therapy.

1. _____

2. _____

3. _____

4. _____

D➤ How long will it take for this woman's symptoms to improve?

_____

ANSWERS/COMMENTS

A➤ Any three of the following: **3**

1. Oral
2. Transdermal
3. Subcutaneous
4. Vaginal

Many candidates have offered the parenteral route. This is too vague as it could refer to patch, gel or implant. A number of candidates have suggested depot injections. Menophase is used in North America but is not available in the UK. The question asked for *common* routes.

B➤ 1. Transdermal   **1**
2. Bypasses liver metabolism and hence may have less effect on   **1**
   clotting mechanism

Fifty percent of candidates have given patch for part 1. The rest have offered a mixture of tablets, implants and creams. While implants bypass liver metabolism, you would not normally use them as a first-line treatment. The advantage offered by transdermal preparations is more theoretical than real but they do not risk lowering the antithrombin III levels. As is often the case, Rose's history is un-certain. A deep vein thrombosis (DVT) was never proven and two subsequent pregnancies were uneventful. Her symptoms are severe and hormone replacement therapy should not be withheld. Vaginal cream will not help this woman's systemic symptoms.

C➤ Any four of the following: **4**

1. Clotting screen
2. Protein C
3. Protein S
4. Antithrombin III
5. Antinuclear factor
6. Complement screen
7. Anticardiolipin antibodies
8. Activated protein C resistance (APCR)

Fifty percent of candidates have given the correct answer. Thrombo-genic screening should be offered to any patient with a history of previous DVT or family history of DVT. Factor V Leiden is only checked if the APCR is abnormal.

ANSWERS/COMMENTS

D➤ 2–3 months

1

Many candidates did not have a clue! Answers varied from seven days to six months. Most said 2–6 weeks. Practitioners must have some idea of when symptomatic relief can be expected to occur so that the patient can be counselled accurately. If no idea of the time scale involved is given, then disillusionment may occur when relief is not immediate, resulting in poor complicance. Vasomotor symptoms respond much sooner than tiredness, poor sleep pattern or vaginal dryness. Topical preparations may be given, in conjunction with systemic regimens, to provide initial relief in the first few months.

QUESTIONS

A 32-year-old patient attends your surgery. Her baby was due ten days ago. She has one previous child which was delivered normally following a spontaneous onset of labour 16 days after her expected date. All her antenatal checks are normal. You perform a vaginal examination and estimate the Bishop's score to be seven.

A➤ What is a Bishop's score?

B➤ What does a score of seven indicate?

C➤ List five factors used to determine the ripeness of the cervix.

1.

2.

3.

4.

5.

D➤ List three separate risks of postmaturity.

1.

2.

3.

ANSWERS/COMMENTS

	Score
	1

A► **A weighted scoring system used when assessing the cervix to estimate how likely it is that the woman will go into labour**

Most candidates have succeeded with this question.

 Howler! A type of partogram.

Bishop's score Cervix	0	1	2
Dilation in cm	0	1–2	3–4
Consistency	Firm	Medium	Soft
Length in cm	>2	1–2	<1
Position	Posterior	Mid	Anterior
Station of foetal head above the ischial spines in cm	3	2	1

B► **Favourable for induction**   1

Twenty percent of candidates have felt that this indicated that the cervix was unripe. Women with a Bishop's score of more than six are considered suitable for induction. Failed induction rates in this group are usually less than 1%.

C► 1. Dilation   1
2. Consistency   1
3. Length   1
4. Position   1
5. Station of the head above the ischial spines   1

Forty percent of candidates have put length of the cervix and effacement as separate functions.

ANSWERS/COMMENTS

D➤ Any three of the following:

Score
3

Risks due to placental insufficiency:

1. Intrauterine death
2. Oligohydramnios
3. Meconium aspirations
4. Foetal distress in labour

Risks due to a big baby:

5. Increased risk of instrumental delivery
6. Risk of shoulder dystocia or cephalopelvic disproportion

A number of candidates have put 'maternal anxiety'. We have a certain sympathy with this answer but did not consider it as a risk in obstetric terms. We did not accept intrauterine death and stillbirth as separate risks.

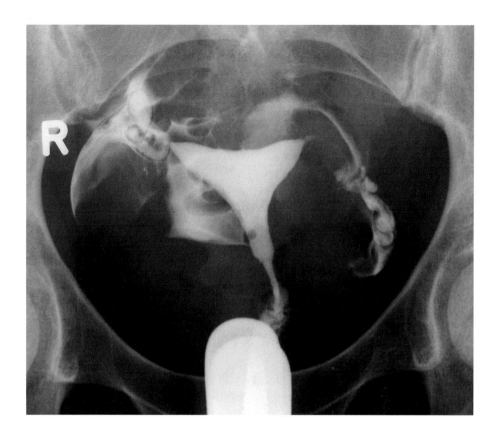

QUESTIONS

Examine the X-ray.

A➤ What is this X-ray called?

_____

B➤ What does it demonstrate?

_____

_____

C➤ At what time in a woman's menstrual cycle should it be performed?

_____

_____

D➤ Is this investigation available to the primary care physician?

Yes/No _____

E➤ List three features this investigation can detect other than tubal problems.

1. _____

2. _____

3. _____

F➤ How would you manage a woman with a history of pelvic infection who is having this investigation?

_____

_____

G➤ What two other investigations, if combined, would provide you with the same information?

1. _____

2. _____

ANSWERS/COMMENTS

	Score

A► **Hysterosalpingogram (HSG)** — 1

B► **Bilateral fill and spill of dye**
Both tubes are open — 1

Despite this being rather obvious, several candidates answered tubal pregnancy or invented tubal stenosis.

C► **The first half after a period, usually within ten days of the onset of menses** — 1

The question asks when in the menstrual cycle you might perform the test; many candidates gave the correct answer. 'Not during a period' is too vague. Mid-cycle (15% of candidates) or secretory phase (13% of candidates) risks performing the test when the woman may be pregnant.

D► **Yes** — 1

Many candidates have fallen into the trap of assuming that the answer was 'no' as the test is not performed in the community. However, a GP can refer a patient directly to the hospital X-ray department without the need to see a specialist in a hospital clinic first.

E► **Any three of the following:** — 3

1. Cervical incompetence
2. Intramural polyp
3. Bicornuate uterus
4. Synechiae
5. Submucous fibroid

This question has been answered quite well, the majority of candidates scoring two marks.

Howler! Vaginal abnormalities.

Pitfall: HSG demonstrates the sequelae of chronic pelvic infection, i.e. tubal blockage, but it does not diagnose pelvic infection itself.

ANSWERS/COMMENTS

Score

F➤ Give antibiotic cover.

1

Many candidates have said that they would take swabs. However, even if the swabs are negative, prophylactic antibiotics should be administered to prevent quiescent infection being reactivated by the HSG.

 Howlers! Postpone test – how long for? Refer for laparoscopy and dye – carries the same risks.

G➤ 1. Hysteroscopy

1

  2. Laparoscopy and dye

1

Most candidates suggested laparoscopy and dye; only 30% answered hysteroscopy. This would be needed to assess the uterine cavity.

REST STATION

INTERACTIVE STATION

Instructions to candidate

You are a local general practitioner qualified for ten years. You are a clinical assistant in the local district hospital where you attend three antenatal clinics a week.

Tracey is 23 years old; this is her first ongoing pregnancy (she had a termination two years ago at eight weeks).

She has a history of intravenous drug abuse. She tended to party a lot and thinks that one of her boyfriends may have been bisexual.

She asked to be tested for HIV as part of her antenatal booking screen. The results have returned positive and it is your job to inform her of the implications of these results.

She is currently 20 weeks pregnant.

Please counsel her accordingly.

Instructions to actress

Tracey is 23 years old. She is fair, slight and rather pale. She has an elfin face. This is her first ongoing pregnancy. She had a termination of pregnancy at eight weeks two years ago.

In her past, when she was a teenager, she 'did' drugs. She started with cannabis and moved on through speed, smack and finally mainline heroin.

She has now kicked the habit and has not used drugs for 18 months. She has a new partner and is looking forward to this planned pregnancy.

She is currently 20 weeks pregnant and because of her past, she asked for HIV testing during her routine booking screen.

Tracey is about to be told that the HIV test is positive. She is about to move through several emotional phases. Firstly disbelief, then anger, guilt and fear. **You will need to demonstrate all these emotions during the interview**.

You are particularly concerned about the effects on your baby and your relationship and will ask the doctor to give you full counselling regarding the implications.

INTERACTIVE STATION

The areas that you should cover are as follows:

- Should I have a termination?
- The effects of pregnancy on HIV
- What are the chances that my baby will be infected too?
- What kind of a birth will I have?
- Should I breast feed?
- Will they take my baby from me?

Instructions to examiner

This station tests the candidate's ability to deal with an emotional patient who has to come to terms with news that will shock and frighten her. The candidate must demonstrate an ability to deal with the patient with sympathy and show an understanding of the emotional onslaught she is suffering. It is also important that the doctor can demonstrate an ability to listen, to direct the interview and to offer accurate medical advice.

ANSWERS/COMMENTS

Marks awarded by the examiner

A➤ Empathy and consideration

0	1	2
No empathy displayed		Very empathetic and considerate of patient's feelings

B➤ Tact and listening skills

0	1	2
Doctor insensitive to patient's needs. Patient continuously interrupted		Patient expectations fully explored. Excellent use of silence and listening

C➤ Well-balanced argument/patient autonomy

0	1	2
Doctor-centred interview. Patient's feelings not explored		Patient fully able to make autonomous decision

D➤ Accuracy of medical facts (including counselling)

0	1	2
Inaccuracy of facts. No counselling offered		Accurate, relevant facts; support counselling offered

Marks awarded by the actress

Felt that doctor knew his/her facts.	1
Would wish to see the doctor again.	1

The basic facts to be included are:

- If the patient is well, research indicates that pregnancy will not affect health.
- Currently the vertical transmission rate is quoted as 20% (some sources say 15%). Of those babies that convert to HIV positive, 50% will develop AIDS.
- HIV infection is not likely to be passed onto the baby during birth, but delivery by caesarean section should be offered.
- During birth, staff will have to take extra care.
- Breast feeding is not recommended at present.

ANSWERS/COMMENTS

- Social workers have a clearly defined brief and that is to support parents and children at home. The child cannot be taken away and put into care simply because one parent is HIV positive.

Wide areas of ignorance were uncovered by this station as demonstrated by the range of marks allocated. Range 1–10, mean 7.5, standard deviation 2.4.

Good candidates were not only offering caesarean section deliveries but also recommending AZT therapy intrapartum to reduce the vertical transmission rate. The European Collaborative Study quotes a 13% vertical transmission rate whereas some American and African studies quote 40%. Fifty percent of vertical transmission is estimated to occur during labour while breast feeding accounts for another 10–20%.

It is of interest that women in the United Kingdom have been identified anonymously as being HIV positive in pregnancy but only 17% of these knew about their HIV infection. There are ethical dilemmas here. Although currently we only test and collect data anonymously the question must be raised as to whether or not the woman has a right to know if she is HIV positive. It would certainly affect her decision to breast feed which has direct implications on vertical transmission rates.

The long-term safety of AZT is still an unresolved issue. Even with a vertical transmission rate of 20%, 80% of infants are destined to be uninfected. We do not have long-term data on AZT toxicity.

Poor candidates unfortunately have fallen into the trap of suggesting termination of pregnancy in this case and some bluntly pointed out to the actress that this was the only ethical thing to do. One candidate demonstrated very little tact and sympathy in stating that as the mother would die very soon anyway there would be very little point in continuing with the pregnancy. In fact, the time scale from presenting with an HIV-positive result to death is approximately 10–12 years.

QUESTIONS

A 37-year-old woman attends your surgery for a routine antenatal visit at 37 weeks' gestation in her third pregnancy. Her previous pregnancies were uncomplicated and deliveries normal. Her booking blood pressure was 130/80. Today her initial blood pressure is 150/100. It settles to 130/90 after ten minutes. She has gained 15 lb since booking and has pitting oedema to her mid-calf. There is a trace of protein on dipsticking her urine. (She has no urinary symptoms.) The fundal height is appropriate for her dates.

A➤ Which of the following would be the most appropriate management for this lady?

1. Refer her for immediate hospital assessment.

   Yes/No
   _____

2. Ask the community midwife to visit her at home the next day.

   Yes/No
   _____

3. Ask her to return to the surgery the following week.

   Yes/No
   _____

B➤ What is the false-positive detection rate for dipsticks when they show a trace of protein?

   %
   _____

QUESTIONS

C➤ Which of the following investigations would you be justified in arranging to further assess this pregnancy?

1. Uric acid.

   Yes/No

2. Midstream urine for microscopy.

   Yes/No

3. Platelet count.

   Yes/No

4. Prothrombin time.

   Yes/No

5. Creatinine.

   Yes/No

D➤ If this woman required antihypertensive medication, which drug would you use?

ANSWERS/COMMENTS

	Score
A➤ 1. No	1
2. Yes	1
3. No	1

Given the history, this woman does not require urgent admission to hospital but you need to increase the antenatal monitoring; 27% of candidates have been prepared to leave Mrs Brown a week, which is too long. The community midwife should attend the next day and recheck the lady's blood pressure and urine analysis in the familiar surroundings of her home.

B➤ **20%**	1

(D) **Differentiator:** *Less than 30% of candidates have answered correctly. Most guessed too low (2–5%).*

	Score
C➤ 1. Yes	1
2. No	1
3. Yes	1
4. No	1
5. No	1

Many candidates have just said yes to everything.

Uric acid and platelet count, if abnormal, would alert you to the fact that Mrs Brown was developing pre-eclampsia. Since it is highly unlikely that the prothrombin time and creatinine would be abnormal, their measurement cannot be justified.

During validation of this question, the need for a midstream urine caused a lot of debate. We feel that in view of Mrs Brown not exhibiting any symptoms and just a trace of protein, this test is not required.

D➤ **Methyldopa or labetolol**	1

Nearly all candidates correctly prescribed methyldopa or labetolol.

QUESTIONS

Study the temperature chart.

A► What does this show?

_____

B► How would you instruct a woman to use it?

1. When does she take her temperature?

_____

2. How does she know she has ovulated?

_____

C► What other physical sign can a woman look for to suggest ovulation?

_____

D► 1. When performing a postcoital test, what day would you do it in a woman with a 28-day cycle?

_____

2. What is a positive postcoital test?

_____

3. Define spinnbarkeit.

_____

E► List three other tests which can be performed to confirm ovulation.

1. _____

2. _____

3. _____

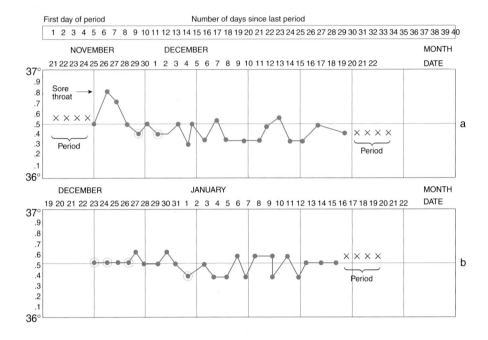

First day of period   Number of days since last period

| 1 | 2 | 3 | 4 | 5 | 6 | 7 | 8 | 9 | 10 | 11 | 12 | 13 | 14 | 15 | 16 | 17 | 18 | 19 | 20 | 21 | 22 | 23 | 24 | 25 | 26 | 27 | 28 | 29 | 30 | 31 | 32 | 33 | 34 | 35 | 36 | 37 | 38 | 39 | 40 |

a

b

ANSWERS/COMMENTS

	Score

A➤ Failure to ovulate   1

Only 50% of candidates have stated anovulation. Most other candidates described the chart.

B➤ 1. First thing in the morning before getting out of bed   1
2. A rise of more than 0.5° around midcycle   1

This has been well answered.

!?! **Howler!** *Temperature goes down.*

C➤ Alteration in cervical mucus which becomes clear   1

✗ **Pitfall:** *Mittelschmerz is a symptom, not a sign. Not every woman has pain midcycle.*

D➤ 1. Day 12–15   1
2. More than five motile sperms in a high-power field   1
3. Length cervical mucus can be drawn from the os   1

1. Most candidates stated that a postcoital test should be performed between days 12 and 14.
2. Most candidates have known that it involves motile sperm but only 15% have given the exact definition.
3. Many candidates have suggested preovulatory thick mucus, others have confused spinnbarkeit with ferning. Overall, this question has been answered poorly.

E➤ Any three of the following: 3

1. Luteal phase progesterone
2. Timed luteal phase endometrial biopsy
3. Follicular tracking with ultrasound
4. Home ovulation kit

!?! **Howler!** *Pregnancy test.*

The role of temperature charts has been called into question by many infertility experts. They do not provide an accurate assessment of ovulation. Most feel they merely increase anxiety. Two or three luteal-phase progesterones (day 21 in a 28-day cycle; day 23 in a 30-day cycle) are used as evidence that ovulation has occurred. However, temperature charts do make good visual questions so do not be surprised to see one in the examination.

QUESTIONS

*Siobhan attends your surgery. She is currently at 38 weeks'
gestation in her third pregnancy which has been completely
uncomplicated to date. She is booked for a home confinement and
wants the third stage of her labour managed in a physiological way.
The midwives are not really keen to do so and asked her to discuss
this with you.*

A➤ What are the three key elements of the physiological management of
the third stage?

1. _____

2. _____

3. _____

B➤ Why are the midwives unhappy?

_____

C➤ List two complications associated with the physiological management of the third stage.

1. _____

2. _____

D➤ What are the two key elements of the active management of the third
stage?

1. _____

2. _____

E➤ List two signs of placental separation.

1. _____

2. _____

ANSWERS/COMMENTS

	Score

A➤ 1. Division of the umbilical cord only when pulsation has ceased   **1**

     2. Delivery of the placenta by maternal effort and aided by gravity without cord traction   **1**

     3. Use of oxytocics only if haemorrhage occurs   **1**

In validation, this question was appallingly answered. We hope you have done better.

Howlers! Mum pulls out the placenta herself; no inversion of the uterus; put baby to the breast; no cutting of the cord at all.

B➤ Risk of complications at home   **1**

Tip: Many candidates have given specific complications but these are needed for question C. Read all the questions and do not give answers to one question if they are required for a subsequent one.

Midwives can cope with emergencies but not at home.

C➤ 1. Postpartum haemorrhage   **1**

     2. Retained placenta   **1**

Retained products, offered by many candidates, is not acceptable. Infection and endometriosis are long-term problems and not specific to the physiological management of the third stage.

D➤ 1. Give syntometrine with delivery of the anterior shoulder.   **1**

     2. Delivery of the placenta by continuous cord traction when separation has occurred   **1**

The accepted answers are quite precise. Many candidates suggested administering syntometrine but they did not specify that it is given with the delivery of the anterior shoulder. A number of candidates wanted to give ergometrine but this is used only if a postpartum haemorrhage occurs.

Howler! Control the uterus.

ANSWERS/COMMENTS

E➤ Any two of the following:

1. Lengthening of the cord
2. Fresh bleeding
3. Uterus contracts, fundus becomes globular

This has been very poorly attempted. Answers have included gush of blood; fundus rising. There is a small trickle of fresh bleeding. The loss should not be heavy.

Howler! Show – a sign of early labour.

Tip: Avoid using abbreviations. For example, you should not use the abbreviation CCT for continuous cord traction. Write all answers in full.

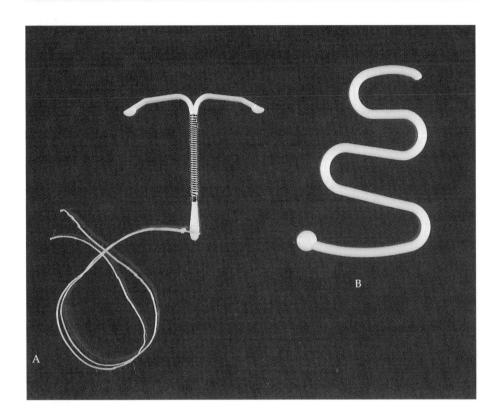

QUESTIONS

Examine the photograph.

A➤ Identify these intrauterine contraceptive devices.

A

B

B➤ What is the principal difference between them?

C➤ List the main mechanism of action of A.

D➤ How long is A effective for?

E➤ At what stage of the menstrual cycle would you normally insert an intrauterine contraceptive device?

F➤ What is the failure rate associated with device A?

G➤ If you regularly insert coils, what first aid equipment must you have on site? (List two examples).

1.

2.

H➤ Following insertion, when should a woman return for a coil check?

ANSWERS/COMMENTS

	Score

A► A **Nova T** — 1

B **Lippe's loop** — 1

Most candidates have identified the Nova T; 50% have had both correct answers.

In 1998 the two most commonly used devices in this country were the Nova T and the Multiload 350. The Mirena is now gaining popularity, but is more expensive. The plastic devices have fallen out of favour. They were suitable for multiparous patients but caused dysmenorrhoea and menorrhagia. Reducing the surface area to minimize side effects reduced efficacy.

B► **Nova T contains copper.** — 1

Only 50% of candidates have given the correct answer.

Howlers! Shape; pre- and postcoital; hormones.

C► **Causes a foreign body reaction on the endometrium, blocking implantation** — 1
or
Copper enhances the foreign body reaction. — 1

A small number of candidates answered that copper reduces sperm motility. This is probably true but this is not its *main* mode of action.

D► **Five years** — 1

E► **During or shortly after a menstrual period** — 1

At validation, only 45% of candidates offered the correct answer. Many put down 'first half of the cycle'. This is too broad as it gives up to day 14 to fit the device. Usually aim for day five of menses.

*Tip: Note the stem asked at what time in the menstrual cycle would a device **normally** be inserted. Obviously, when used for postcoital contraception, the coil can be inserted up to day 19 of a 28-day cycle, i.e. five days after ovulation.*

ANSWERS/COMMENTS

F➤ 1–2 per 100 woman-years

Many underestimated the failure rate.

The Ortho-Gynae T Slimline 380 copper intrauterine contraceptive device has been available for a number of years and is, surprisingly, infrequently used. It is effective for at least eight years, it is cheap and the additional copper collars on the transverse side arms increase its efficacy to 0.3 per 100 woman-years. This is as effective as the oral combined contraceptive pill.

G➤ Any two of the following:

1. Adrenaline 1 ml of 1:1000 for subcutaneous injection
2. Oxygen
3. A Brook airway
4. Diazepam 10 mg for intravenous injection
5. Atropine 0.6 mg for intravenous injection

When validating this section, lots of answers were provided but, obviously, we wanted the key therapy needed to save life, not miscellaneous factors such as good light, firm couch, syringe and needles, etc.

The main complications of IUD insertion that can occasionally occur are:

- Persistent bradycardia, treated with atropine if pulse is persistently less than 60 beats per minute
- Cardiac arrest
- Asthmatic attack or allergic reaction, treated with adrenaline
- Grand mal attack. This can occur in the absence of any history of epilepsy or of any subsequent fits. It is usually self-limiting but diazepam should be available.

Beware of vomiting and consequent inhalation of fluid when consciousness returns.

H➤ After next period (4–6 weeks)

This question has been poorly answered. Many candidates have suggested 6–12 weeks.

QUESTIONS

Mrs Brown attended for booking last week, having just recently moved into the area. She was 28 weeks pregnant. The midwife asks you to look at her booking blood results.

White blood cells	7.4×10^9 (4.0–11)
Haemoglobin	8 g/dl (11.5–14)
MCV	70 FL (76–96)
MCH	25 µg (27–32)
MCHC	29% (30–35)

A➤ What is the most likely diagnosis?

B➤ What other two investigations would you perform?

1.

2.

C➤ 1. Is there any other condition which might give you the same blood picture?

2. How could you exclude this?

QUESTIONS

D➤ Assuming the most likely diagnosis, would you:

1. give jectofer?

   Yes/No

2. give folic acid 5 mg/day?

   Yes/No

3. perform a bone marrow biopsy?

   Yes/No

4. give a blood transfusion?

   Yes/No

5. advise against breast feeding?

   Yes/No

ANSWERS/COMMENTS

Score

A► **Iron deficiency anaemia**   1

All individuals have answered this correctly.

B► 1. Ferritin levels   1
2. Total iron-binding capacity   1

Mostly, this question has been well answered. There have been some
odd answers offered, for example haemoglobin electrophoresis. This
is not relevant if iron-deficient anaemia is the diagnosis. Also, reticu-
locyte count has been offered. This indicates the response to iron
therapy; it is hardly relevant as a diagnostic investigation.

C► 1. β Thalassaemia   1
2. Haemoglobin electrophoresis   1

1. Quite a mixture of answers have been offered including sickle cell
   disease (20%) and megaloblastic anaemia (10%).

   ☞ *Tip: One or two candidates have given haemoglobin electrophoresis – this is a test. Therefore it should not be offered as an
   answer to a question asking for a condition.*

2. Quite a mixture of answers have been offered but only 50% were
   correct.

D► 1. No   1
2. No   1
3. No   1
4. No   1
5. No   1

Blood transfusion is too aggressive an intervention at 28 weeks. There
is plenty of time to get a response to iron before delivery. Jectofer is
invasive with side effects, i.e. a sore injection site and a slight risk of
anaphylaxis. As a working rule, allow one week for iron to be
absorbed into the marrow and then a rise of 1 g per week thereafter.

Surprisingly, many candidates wanted to prescribe folate.

INTERACTIVE STATION

Instructions to candidate

This is a consultation between yourself and Mrs Judge, a 47-year-old with two children aged 16 and 18 years who works as a beauty consultant.

She has suffered terrible menorrhagia resulting in anaemia in the last two years and has required iron therapy. She has finally decided to go ahead with a hysterectomy after failure of medical treatment. She attended her local hospital gynaecological outpatient department last week where she was seen by the registrar and given a date for admission for total abdominal hysterectomy and bilateral salpingo-oophorectomy.

She is still quite uneasy about the prospect of surgery and has made an appointment to see you today.

Instructions to actress

You are Mrs Judge, a 47-year-old mother of two teenage children aged 16 and 18 years. You work as a beauty consultant and have always prided yourself on being well turned out with good colour co-ordination and make-up. You work out in a gymnasium twice a week.

You have suffered severe menorrhagia for two years and have become quite anaemic. Your doctor prescribed iron and the local gynaecological outpatient department has tried several different preparations to try to control the blood loss. Nothing has proved successful and you were seen last week in the hospital clinic and given a date for an abdominal hysterectomy.

You are concerned about a number of issues which you wish to discuss with your doctor, who you feel knows you better than the gynaecological team.

- You have not really come to terms with the thought of losing your womb and regard this as a loss of femininity.
- You are most concerned that they will remove your ovaries as well and this will result in a premature menopause and ageing.
- Equally, you fear HRT as a measure for preventing premature menopause and ageing.
- You are worried that after the hysterectomy you will put on weight.
- You look for reassurance that you won't be depressed after surgery.
- You are concerned about the effect a hysterectomy might have on your sex life.

ANSWERS/COMMENTS

Marks awarded by the examiner

A➤ Sympathy

0	1	2
Poor sympathy shown		Very sensitive and sympathetic

B➤ Listening skills

0	1	2
Poor listener – talked over patient		Good listener – allowed patient to express her views

C➤ Counselling skills

0	1	2
Poor counselling, no support group offered, topics poorly covered		Good counselling, hysterectomy support offered, all topics covered well

D➤ Knowledge base

0	1	2
Poor knowledge of effects of hysterectomy, arguments for and against oophorectomy and facts of HRT		Good knowledge of effects of operation, arguments re oophorectomy and facts on HRT

Marks awarded by the actress

Comfortable with doctor/would see this person again	0/1
Doctor/knew what he/she was talking about	0/1

Discussion to include:

- Reassurance re femininity, i.e. good wife and mother/looks after herself/womb no longer needed now as family complete and is affecting her health and quality of life/'femininity is from within'.
- Pose arguments for and against removal of ovaries. Ultimately if there is no sign of disease the choice should be made by the patient, but she can only make an informed choice with accurate information: 15–20% of ovaries cease functioning early after surgery even if conserved/ increased risk of ovarian cancer in the 50s (a silent killer – no national screening programme and often presents late)/we are obviously taking out more ovaries than we need to but no predictor test available to help us decide who is at risk. Gene marker test for ovarian cancer is only available if there is a strong family history.

ANSWERS/COMMENTS

- HRT helps protect against osteoporosis and ischaemic heart disease, high cholesterol and Alzheimer's dementia (recent studies). It does not cause weight gain. Two extra cases of breast cancer per 1000 women on HRT for 5 years. Six extra cases of breast cancer per 1000 women on HRT for 10 years.
- Depression and weight gain post-hysterectomy are old wives tales, but it is true that depression is more likely to occur if the patient has not come to terms with the surgery before it is performed.
- Sex should still be good. There no longer will be cervical excitation if a total hysterectomy is performed, but vaginal capacity is preserved and clitoral stimulation is still possible.

Allocation of marks using the RCOG format:

From the actress

Appropriate eye contact	1
Listened attentively	1
Confidence in candidate	1
I would like to see this person again.	1

From the examiner

Introduction	1
Put patient at ease	1
Avoidance of medical jargon	1
Explanation of condition	1
Verbal clues followed	1
Non-verbal clues followed	1

The examiner will be looking for a good explanation of the facts regarding hysterectomy, a good, well-balanced argument for whether the ovaries should be removed or not and a pleasant manner.

We have been rather surprised that this station has not been better attempted. Although the average mark was good, the range was quite wide and some candidates demonstrated a surprising lack of knowledge about a basic gynaecological procedure. Range 5–10, mean 8.2, standard deviation 1.2.

We include two possible marking systems here:

1. One we used to validate the station, allowing freedom to demonstrate a range of interactive skills and knowledge.
2. The other is one of the RCOG formats.

REST STATION

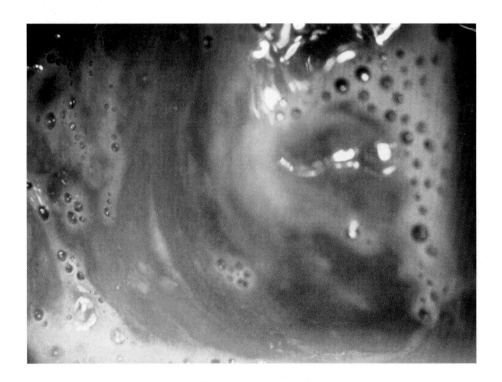

QUESTIONS

A➤ Study the photograph in front of you. What is the most common cause of abnormal vaginal discharge?

_____

B➤ 1. If your patient has *Candida*, you must always treat the male partner.

True/False
_____

2. Candida infections are not related to the use of the combined oral contraceptive pill.

True/False
_____

3. The male is vector for trichomonal infections.

True/False
_____

4. Menopausal women are often asymptomatic carriers for *Trichomonas*.

True/False
_____

C➤ Bacterial vaginosis:

1. carries a five- to sevenfold increased risk for late miscarriage or preterm labour.

True/False
_____

2. is associated with vaginal cuff cellulitis following vaginal hysterectomy.

True/False
_____

3. untreated, increases the risk of endometritis after termination of pregnancy, even in asymptomatic carriers.

True/False
_____

4. May act as a co-factor to human papilloma virus in the pathogenesis of cervical dysplasia.

True/False
_____

D➤ What kind of organism is *Trichomonas vaginalis*?

_____

ANSWERS/COMMENTS

	Score

A► Bacterial vaginosis   1

Fifty percent of candidates have identified bacterial vaginosis correctly from the photograph. Many people gave an answer of *Candida*
and a few *Trichomonas* and one *Gardnerella*.

B► 1. False   1
2. False   1
3. True   1
4. True   1

1. Even if the male partner was thought to be the vector for *Candida*
   the answer would still be false.

    *Tip: The stem contains the word **always**. Virtually nothing is
   always true – the male partner could be using the sheath which
   would act as protection against infection.*

Almost two thirds of the candidates have given incorrect answers to
parts 2 and 4. Menopausal women are often asymptomatic carriers
for a number of infections since atrophic vaginitis does predispose to
infections.

C► 1. True   1
2. True   1
3. True   1
4. True   1

Only 12.5% of candidates have had all four parts correct. The majority had three out of four correct.

D► Protozoan (flagellate protozoan)   1

Some candidates felt that *Trichomonas* was an anaerobic Gram-
negative organism. Certainly suggesting 'obligate intracellular para-
site' does not answer the question that was asked.

QUESTIONS

A directive from the Department of Health has stated that 'all women should have the opportunity antenatally to be involved in constructing a birth plan'.

A➤ What are the two most important functions of a birth plan?

1. _____

2. _____

B➤ List six important areas that should be covered by a birth plan.

1. _____

2. _____

3. _____

4. _____

5. _____

6. _____

C➤ How could this be monitored?

1. _____

2. _____

ANSWERS/COMMENTS

	Score

A► 1. To address maternal expectations   **1**

2. To act as a formal basis of discussion between health care   **1**
professionals

The majority of candidates have had a good feel for this question. Flexibility, the woman's choice and women in control were the key issues. A number of candidates, however, raised areas not covered by birth plans, including discussion of home versus hospital confinement and the opportunity to reinforce health education.

B► Any six of the following: **6**

1. Foetal monitoring
2. Ambulation during labour
3. Pain relief
4. Disposal of placenta
5. Cord clamping
6. Delivery position
7. Who is present (medical students, etc.)
8. Episiotomy . . . or not
9. Vitamin K . . . or not
10. Length of stay

The majority of candidates have scored four or five marks. Topics such as antenatal tests and site of delivery are not areas covered in birth plans.

C► 1. Quality control audit   **1**

2. Patient satisfaction audit   **1**

This section has been answered poorly. Only 25% of candidates included the term 'audit' in their answers. Quality control allows the provider unit to assess how well they are meeting the expressed needs of their clients. Patient satisfaction questionnaires allow the clients to give their views of the service provided.

QUESTIONS

Score

You are asked to see a baby with conjunctivitis (not just sticky eyes).

A➤ If the baby is four days old:

1. what is the most likely diagnosis?

2. what initial treatment would you recommend?

3. If the symptoms failed to settle, what antibiotic drug would you use?

B➤ If the baby is eight days old and has failed to respond to the above treatment:

1. what is the most likely diagnosis?

2. how would you confirm the diagnosis?

3. what treatment would you use?

C➤ What other two important measures should be undertaken in the second case?

1.

2.

ANSWERS/COMMENTS

	Score

A➤ 1. Staphylococcal conjunctivitis   **2**
   2. Neomycin eye drops   **1**
   3. Flucloxacillin   **1**

1. A very poor attempt to answer a question relating to a common neonatal problem. The stem asked for the 'most likely diagnosis'. Approximately 30% of candidates were correct. Gonococcal conjunctivitis is hardly the most common cause for sticky eyes in a neonate four days old.

 Tip: Read the question. Bacterial conjunctivitis is too non-specific.

Other offerings included *Haemophilus influenzae* and *Streptococcus pneumoniae*.

2. We were a little unsure what the candidate who answered 'breast milk' was intending here. However, several midwifery colleagues and health visitors do in fact advocate the use of breast milk here, as it is sterile, cheap and plentiful.

   Approximately 60% of candidates gave saline bathing as the answer. Having piloted this question three times now, there has certainly been controversy over the answer. This question was also piloted in the entire paediatric department of one author's hospital to avoid local bias, as every unit has its own protocol. Many of the paediatric junior staff had been trained elsewhere. Saline bathing is now considered rather out of date.

3. Several candidates gave penicillin as the answer. Flucloxacillin is a better choice for staphylococcal infections. Chloramphenicol was the most popular response.

B➤ 1. *Chlamydia*   **2**
   2. Chlamydial corneal scrapes   **1**
   3. Tetracycline eye drops and erythomycin orally for 14 days   **1**

1. The majority were correct with *Chlamydia*. One or two still considered gonococcal infection as more likely, but not at eight days of age.
2. Very few candidates were specific enough, giving 'eye swabs' as the answer. Immunoassay and Gram staining were among the other attempts.
3. Even when the correct diagnosis was given, the treatment was usually wrong. Obviously, candidates who put *Gonococcus* for part

ANSWERS/COMMENTS

1 had all three parts incorrect. Only one candidate considered tetracycline eye drops in conjunction with oral erythromycin, although several offered the latter alone. Neomycin, cyrofloxacin and flucloxacillin were among the wrong answers.

C➤ Any two of the following:

2

1. Parental referral to GUM clinic for screening and/or therapy
2. Review infant after 14 days to ensure resolution and also that infant has not developed systemic signs, especially pneumonia.
3. Notifiable disease

There were very few correct answers here. Many candidates suggested screening and treating the mother and forgot the partner.

One candidate sadly gave one incorrect answer and offered 'chest X-ray and treat the mother' as the second answer. Though both were covered, this candidate would only receive one mark.

 Tip: Do put each answer on a separate line to receive full marks; never put two answers against one slot. Similarly, some candidates put 'screen the mother' as one answer and 'screen the partner' as the second. This wasted a potential mark.

QUESTIONS

Score

A➤ Urinary symptoms are common in women _____ %
experience at least one episode a year.

(Please insert the correct answer: 25%, 40%, 60%, 75%)

B➤ What percentage of symptomatic women have no significant bacterial growth on urine culture?

_____ %

C➤ Name four infective causes of dysuria associated with a sterile midstream urine culture.

1. _____

2. _____

3. _____

4. _____

D➤ Name three non-infective causes of frequency and urgency.

1. _____

2. _____

3. _____

E➤ Asymptomatic bacteriuria can occur in 10% of pregnant women. What percentage of these will develop ascending pyelonephritis if left untreated?

_____ %

ANSWERS/COMMENTS

A➤ 25%

1

Urinary tract infections are a common problem in women and frequently present to the general practitioner's surgery. Yet on the whole, this question was poorly answered.

 Differentiator: *Just under 20% of candidates were correct for question A. The majority felt more women had problems and the most quoted answer was 40%.*

B➤ 30–50%

1

Similarly, just under half the candidates were correct with question B. There are many reasons why a patient may present with symptoms and yet no growth is detected on a midstream urine culture. Firstly, frequency and urgency are very non-specific symptoms (see answer to question D) and do not always indicate infection. Secondly, specimens are often left in the refrigerator overnight and are not plated out as fresh specimens. Lastly, dysuria can be due to a number of conditions (see answers to question C) other than bacterial infections.

C➤ Any four of the following:

4

1. *Chlamydia* ⎫ Cause 'internal' dysuria. i.e. true
2. Gonorrhea ⎭ urethritis
3. Herpes simplex ⎫ Cause 'external' dysuria, i.e. vulvitis
4. *Trichomonas vaginalis* ⎪ +/– ulceration
5. *Candida albicans* ⎬ Occasionally *Trichomonas* can be
6. TB ⎭ isolated from the urinary tract

A depressing number of candidates gave bacterial causes of infection as answers to question C, despite the fact that the stem said *sterile* midstream urine culture. Only 16% were correct.

ANSWERS/COMMENTS

D➤ Any three of the following:

1. Interstitial cystitis
2. Urethral syndrome
3. Atrophic urethritis and trigonitis
4. Postradiation cystitis
5. Carcinoma
6. Detrusor instability
7. Diabetes

Question D was appallingly answered. At validation, many candidates offered lower motor neurone disease and multiple sclerosis. *Both* are causes of detrusor instability. One would be accepted and score a mark, but both would not be as the same answer is, in effect, being counted twice.

Some candidates suggested genuine stress incontinence as a cause of frequency and urgency. Here they are demonstrating confusion over the compensation techniques some ladies employ. Ladies with bladder neck weakness void frequently, mainly because they know they will minimize leakage if the bladder is kept relatively empty. However, these women would not exhibit urgency.

E➤ 20–30%

A third of the candidates were correct on the last question.

QUESTIONS

Mrs Shah attends your surgery complaining of continual nausea and vomiting. She is now nine weeks by dates, in her first pregnancy.

A➤ Name two investigations you would perform and why.

1. _____

2. _____

B➤ What initial basic home management would you recommend (list three actions)?

1. _____

2. _____

3. _____

C➤ What criteria would you use to decide if hospital admission is necessary?

_____

_____

D➤ Mrs Shah is still in hospital after two weeks and you visit her on the ward. She is still unhappy and unresponsive to therapy. What may this imply?

_____

_____

_____

E➤ Prochloroperazine is:

a   a potent phenothiazine neuroleptic.

True/False

b   excreted in breast milk.

True/False

c   a neuroleptic that may occasionally prolong labour.

True/False

ANSWERS/COMMENTS

Score

A➤ 1. MSU to exclude UTI   1
2. Ultrasound to exclude mole or twins   1

Hyperemesis is another common problem, which can sometimes be difficult to treat. Urinary tract infections, molar and, of course, multiple pregnancies are all associated with increased nausea and vomiting, the latter two because of raised human chorionic gonadotrophin levels. Often simple measures are the best. Hyperemesis should be taken seriously, however. If severe and unresolved, Wernicke's encephalopathy (due to B_1 deficiency) and pontine myelinosis (due to sodium depletion) may result.

B➤ Any three of the following: 3

1. Reassurance
2. Small regular meals
3. Avoid spicy food.
4. Rehydrate
5. Avoid drugs if possible.

This question clearly wanted a practical response to management in the primary care setting. Many candidates offered approaches that were too interventional, such as 'put up a drip, insert nasogastric tube', etc. Rehydration is probably the key to breaking the vicious circle and, obviously, avoidance of spicy foods is good advice in this particular case. Once hospitalized, randomized trials have shown that antiemetics, antihistimines, H_2 receptor blockers and root ginger all help.

C➤ Prolonged vomiting with inability to keep down fluids, together with: 1

Ketosis, on urinalysis
or
Deranged urea and electrolytes and liver function tests
or
Profound weight loss

This question asked for criteria that would be used to decide whether or not to admit to hospital. This reinforced the message that question B was alluding to care in the surgery and at home.

 Tip: Read right through the station before diving in and attempting a stem.

ANSWERS/COMMENTS

Score

D➤ Is there any underlying social or domestic conflict? Does she have problems at home? Is she under pressure to have a termination of pregnancy?

1

Prolonged hyperemesis despite adequate therapy (rehydration and antiemetics) and in the absence of predisposing factors or recurrent admissions does suggest underlying stress and conflict. It is often prevalent in minority and immigrant communities where the patient may feel alone and isolated. Arranged marriages and the extended family, i.e. no privacy for the young couple, may be factors in some cases.

In some situations the woman would prefer a termination but does not wish to say so openly. She may continue to exhibit symptoms whilst asking if the pregnancy is alright or if the vomiting is harming the foetus. She may wish to be told that a termination would be best, as this takes away the personal element of guilt. Psychosomatic factors must be adequately explored.

E➤ 1. a True

1

    b True

1

  2. True

1

 Differentiator: *This is a commonly prescribed drug so some facts should be known. Most candidates scored one, 40% scored two. Remember, only a score of seven out of ten is needed on each station for security and most of this station was very straightforward.*

STRUCTURED ORAL

Information to candidate

Mrs Mitchell is 40 years old and a mother of three. A recent cervical smear report showed 'dense sheets of darkly staining malignant cells' and you referred her for urgent colposcopy to the local hospital. She has booked an emergency appointment to see you today and enters your room looking very distressed.

Instructions to examiner

You are to take the part of Mrs Mitchell, a 40-year-old mother of three.

A➤ Mrs Mitchell: 'Doctor, I had to see you today, I'm still shaking. You know that at the colposcopy appointment the doctor looked very concerned and brought me in straight away for an examination and biopsies under anaesthetic? Well, I went back for the results yesterday and it's CANCER! He kept saying it was a good cell type and it was at the first stage . . . Stage 1. He said it was hopeful. What does all this mean?' (Answer to include description of differentiation and staging for two marks.)

Candidate:

B➤ Mrs Mitchell: They want to operate! They said radiotherapy gives just as good results, but that surgery was better for me. Why? (Expect two reasons for two marks.)

Candidate:

C➤ Mrs Mitchell: Well, I'm confused. Everyone says surgery is better – but then they say I might need radiotherapy afterwards anyway! Why, if surgery is better? (One mark)

Candidate:

D➤ Mrs Mitchell: How long will I be in hospital if I do have surgery? (One mark)

Candidate:

E➤ Mrs Mitchell: The surgeon said he was going to refer me to one of his colleagues who does this sort of operation more often. He said in experienced hands, complications were minimal. What complications are we talking about in the short and long term? (Candidate to name four complications, at least one of which must be long term.)

Candidate:

ANSWERS/COMMENTS

	Score

You are scored for the accuracy of the factual content of your replies.

A➤ Answer to include description of differentiation and staging. Stage 1 – invasive carcinoma confined to the cervix.   **2**

B➤ She is 40 years old. Surgery allows any two of the following: **2**

1. Preservation of the ovaries.
2. Better preservation of sexual function (vaginal stenosis occurs in up to 85% of irradiated patients unless topical oestrogens are applied).
3. A more accurate prognosis can be obtained (i.e. nodal sampling). Total staging is not possible from an examination under anaesthetic.

C➤ You need to explain that we think the growth is confined to the cervix but only when we have examined the nodes will we know for sure. If the nodes are involved, radiotherapy will be necessary.   **1**

D➤ Usually 2–3 weeks   **1**

E➤ We expect four complications as a minimum to be discussed, at least one of which must be in the long-term category.   **4**

Short-term and intermediate complications:
1. Haemorrhage
2. Shock
3. Sepsis
4. Thrombosis

Long-term complications:
1. Ureteric and rectal fistulae
2. Bladder dysfunction
3. Lymphocyst formation

 Differentiator: *Most candidates had a good feel of the meaning of Stage 1 carcinoma of the cervix and were able to reassure Mrs Mitchell on this.*

Some had surprisingly little idea of the basic concept of staging, which was relevant to both the first and second questions. An examination under anaesthestic is necessary to assess the mobility of the cervix and whether or not there is spread into the paracervical tissues. Cystoscopy is often performed at the same time to exclude anterior extension into the bladder base. This basic examination will give the clinician some idea of whether surgery is possible or not.

ANSWERS/COMMENTS

Usually a Wertheim's hysterectomy is reserved for stage Ib and, possibly, IIa tumours. More extensive growths do not do well with surgery and radiotherapy is a more realistic option, with about the same five-year survival rates. However, complete staging requires surgery for pelvic node sampling.

The option of surgery is especially relevant to young, sexually active patients. Vaginal stenosis was a common sequela to radiotherapy until the application of topical oestrogens was introduced, when the incidence dropped to 30%.

Preservation of the ovaries is highly relevant although, of course, if full postoperative histology confirms node involvement then postoperative radiotherapy becomes necessary and will ablate ovarian function. This latter category represents a group of 'forgotten women' who frequently fail to receive the hormone replacement therapy they now need.

The advantages of surgery in the younger group of patients were poorly understood.

Again, some candidates had difficulty with handling this situation and were poor at describing medical information in lay terms and demonstrating sensitivity at the same time. As this was a structured oral, with the examiner taking on the patient role, this was not too important. The station was designed primarily to test knowledge. It could, however, easily be restructured to allow Mrs Mitchell's dilemma to be treated as an interactive station when tact, diplomacy and communication skills are all important.

Most candidates were able to offer short-term complications but few had any knowledge of the specific long-term complications related to Wertheim's hysterectomy or their rate of incidence. These are important facts to include when counselling a patient. Radiotherapy may also cause some bladder dysfunction, chiefly frequency and dysuria. Bladder ulcers can occur. Vesicovaginal fistulae are rare, occurring 3–8 months after treatment. Ureterovaginal fistulae are more likely to occur if surgery and radiotherapy are combined.

Multiple choice questions

QUESTIONS

1➤ Mechanisms of labour in a primigravida

A During the first stage, the uterine muscle contracts and retracts.

B The cervix becomes effaced during the latent phase.

C The average length of the first stage is 12 hours.

D Voluntary effort is essential during the second stage to achieve a spontaneous vaginal delivery.

E Braxton Hicks contractions do not occur before 36 weeks.

2➤ Placenta praevia is more commonly associated with

A Twin pregnancy.

B Previous lower segment caesarean section.

C Face presentation.

D Previous manual removal of placenta.

E Multiparity.

3➤ Urinary tract infection during pregnancy

A Occurs in 1–2% of pregnancies.

B Is diagnosed by finding more than 10 000 bacteria / ml on culture.

C Should have an ultrasound of the renal tract performed.

D Is more common in primigravidae.

E Is a cause of preterm labour.

4➤ High-risk features for abnormal glucose tolerance in pregnancy include

A Maternal weight more than 100 kg at booking.

B Paternal first-degree relative with diabetes.

C Foetal microsomia on ultrasound.

D Single episode of glycosuria at 36 weeks.

E Presence of oligohydramnios.

5➤ All pregnant women are still screened for syphilis

A The Venereal Disease Research Laboratory (VDRL) slide test is a specific serological test.

B The VDRL test remains positive for ever once the mother has been infected.

C Congenital syphilis causes skeletal damage to the neonate.

D Treatment of syphilis in early pregnancy will not protect the foetus.

E Untreated syphilis may result in prematurity.

6► **The placenta acts as an efficient barrier against most infection in the mother, but the following may cross the placenta**

A Neisseria gonorrhoeae.

B Cytomegalovirus.

C Herpes genitalis.

D Parvovirus.

E Toxoplasmosis.

7► **Binovular twins**

A May occur as a result of fertilization of a single ovum.

B Are more common in women under the age of 35 years.

C Are more common in tall women.

D Have a separate chorion and amnion.

E Are at increased risk of twin–twin transfusion.

8► **Maternal mortality**

A Is defined as the death of a woman associated with pregnancy or with childbirth within 28 days of that event.

B In England the incidence is 8.6 per 10 000 births.

C The most common cause is haemorrhage.

D Includes deaths associated with therapeutic termination.

E The majority of anaesthetic deaths in the last triannual report were associated with epidurals.

9► **Pulmonary embolism**

A Is the commonest cause of maternal death.

B Three quarters occur following delivery.

C Is more common following an operative delivery.

D Is preceded by signs of a deep venous thrombosis in the majority of cases.

E A ventilation–perfusion scan is contraindicated during pregnancy.

10► **Breast feeding**

A Most of the feed is obtained within the first five minutes.

B A set regime of feeding should be encouraged.

C Provides the baby with anti-infective agents.

D Should be abandoned if lactation is insufficient during the first week.

E Is contraindicated in the presence of inverted nipples.

QUESTIONS

11► Nerve plexus damage

A Erb's palsy is caused by damage to the roots of the brachial plexus C7 and C8.

B Erb's palsy is associated with the waiter tip deformity.

C If recovery occurs within six months, it is usually complete.

D Erb's palsy is usually associated with hyperextension of the arm during a difficult breech delivery.

E A facial palsy caused by forcep blades usually recovers within a few weeks.

12► Congenital dislocation of the hips

A Is more common among boys.

B Is associated with breech presentation.

C Is best diagnosed using ultrasound.

D If splinted, will be successfully treated after three months.

E Will require surgical correction in 15% of cases.

13► During a normal pregnancy

A Women require an additional 100 kcal a day to ensure normal growth of the foetus.

B Most women's haemoglobin level will fall by 1 g/dl due to haemodilution.

C About 10% of dietary iron is absorbed.

D 300 μg of folic acid is required a day.

E Iron should be given with meals as it is only absorbed in the ferric state and this is best achieved in the presence of vitamin C.

14► Confirmation of pregnancy

A Enzyme-linked immunosorbent assays (ELISA) can confirm a pregnancy before the first missed period.

B Using an abdominal probe, a foetal heart can be seen at six weeks.

C ELISA test is usually performed using maternal blood.

D The uterus is palpable per abdomen at 12 weeks' gestation.

E The α subunit of human chorionic gonadotrophin is immunologically specific.

15► Twin pregnancies are associated with

A An increased incidence of pre-eclampsia.

B Folic acid deficiency.

C Maternal age of more than 35 years.

D An increased incidence of retained placenta.

E Abruptio placentae.

16➤ The incidence of placental abruption is increased with

A External cephalic version.

B Multiparity.

C Threatened miscarriage early in the pregnancy.

D Prolonged labour.

E Raised maternal serum α-fetoprotein.

17➤ Recognized causes of spontaneous preterm labour include

A Polyhydramnios.

B Pre-eclampsia.

C Previous caesarean section.

D Gestational diabetes.

E Pyelonephritis.

18➤ In cases of premature rupture of the membranes, chorioamnionitis should be suspected if

A The maternal white cell count rises.

B A maternal pyrexia occurs.

C Liquor stops draining.

D Foetal movements increase.

E The foetal heart becomes tachycardic.

19➤ Prolapse of the umbilical cord

A Complicates one in 1000 deliveries.

B Is more common with a brow presentation.

C Is associated with spasm of the umbilical arteries from cooling.

D Occurring at home is an indication to call the flying squad.

E Never occurs in a primigravida.

20➤ Physiology of pregnancy

A Cardiac output increases by up to 40%.

B A systolic injection murmur can occur.

C Glomerular filtration rate decreases by 40%.

D The vital capacity of the lungs rises towards term.

E Hypochlorhydria occurs because of regurgitation of alkaline chyle from the intestine.

21► The following drugs, if taken regularly by a lactating woman, may have clinically detectable effects on the neonate

A Diazepam.

B Lithium carbonate.

C Carbimazole.

D Warfarin sodium.

E Tricyclic antidepressants.

22► Recognized complications of delivery at 32 weeks

A Transient tachypnoea.

B Poor temperature control.

C Meconium aspiration syndrome.

D Apnoeic attacks.

E Jaundice.

23► Oligohydramnios is characteristically associated with

A Diabetes mellitus.

B Postmaturity syndrome.

C Rhesus isoimmunization.

D Foetal renal agenesis.

E Oesophageal atresia.

24► External cephalic version

A Should not be performed if the breech presentation is footling.

B May lead to foetal bradycardia.

C Requires a general anaesthetic.

D Is a recognized cause of transplacental haemorrhage.

E Should not be performed before 34 weeks.

25► Recognized causes of vomiting in the second trimester of pregnancy include

A Ectopic pregnancy.

B Hydatidiform mole.

C Ulcerative colitis.

D Acute pyelonephritis.

E Maternal age over 40 years.

QUESTIONS

26► Transcervical biopsy of the chorionic villus

- A Can be used to diagnose neural tube defects earlier than an amniocentesis.
- B Limb deformities are a recognized complication.
- C The associated miscarriage risk is lower than with amniocentesis.
- D If the procedure fails, performing an amniocentesis is contraindicated.
- E Is associated with a 10% risk of placental mosaicism.

27► Bicornuate uterus is associated with an increased risk of

- A Polyhydramnios.
- B Retained placenta.
- C Cervical incompetence.
- D Unstable lie.
- E Prolonged labour.

28► Babies born to diabetic mothers are more at risk of

- A Shoulder dystocia at delivery.
- B Respiratory distress syndrome.
- C Neonatal anaemia.
- D Neonatal hyperglycaemia.
- E Neonatal hypothermia.

29► Breech presentation at 38 weeks' gestation

- A Complicates 3% of all labours.
- B 40% will be a frank or extended breech.
- C Is associated with higher risk of foetal abnormality.
- D May be associated with a uterine abnormality.
- E More commonly presents as a footling breech in primigravidae.

30► The following are sex-linked disorders

- A Ehlers–Danlos syndrome.
- B Spherocytosis.
- C Duchenne muscular dystrophy.
- D Achondroplasia.
- E Hunter mucopolysaccharidosis.

31► Expulsion of an intrauterine contraceptive device

- A Occurs within the first three months in the majority of cases.
- B Is more common among young women.
- C Is more common in multiparous women.
- D If suspected, the woman should be referred for a pelvic ultrasound.
- E Is a contraindication to fitting a further device.

QUESTIONS

32➤ The following drugs inhibit spermatogenesis

A Antimalarials.

B Nitrofurantoin.

C Methyldopa.

D Sulphasalazine.

E Monoamine oxidase inhibitors.

33➤ The natural defence mechanism of the lower genital tract includes

A Bacteriostatic effect of the cervical mucus.

B The high pH of cervical secretions.

C Apposition of the labia and vaginal walls.

D Natural resistance of stratified squamous epithelium.

E Regular menstruation.

34➤ Septic abortion

A *E. coli* is one of the commonest infective organisms.

B Infection is confined to the decidua in 80% of cases.

C Requires urgent evacuation of the uterus as first-line management.

D May lead to long-term infertility.

E Rarely occurs before 12 weeks' gestation.

35➤ Endometrial ablation

A May be performed using a laser.

B Produces amenorrhoea in 90% of cases.

C May be used as a method of sterilization.

D Should not be performed in women with a past history of pelvic inflammatory disease.

E May be performed as a day case.

36➤ Hyperemesis gravidarum requiring hospital admission

A Rarely occurs before nine weeks' gestation.

B Occurs in one in 1000 pregnancies in the UK.

C Is more common in molar pregnancies.

D May require therapeutic termination of pregnancy.

E May lead to thiamine deficiency.

QUESTIONS

37► **In the management of a patient with terminal cervical cancer**

    A Pethidine is the analgesia of choice.

    B Prednisolone 20 mg a day will increase appetite and a sense of well-being.

    C Palliative radiotherapy is indicated to arrest heavy bleeding from the cervix.

    D Constipation may be related to opiate use.

    E Lymphoedema is a common problem.

38► **The urethral syndrome**

    A Significant bacteriuria is present in only half of the cases of urethral syndrome.

    B Is more common before the menopause.

    C Detrusor instability is present in over 25% of cases.

    D May be the first symptom in multiple sclerosis.

    E May be helped by sodium bicarbonate.

39► **Cervical incompetence**

    A Is a common cause of first trimester abortions.

    B Can only be diagnosed by clinical history.

    C Commonly occurs following large loop excision of the transformation zone.

    D Requires a cervical circlage before ten weeks' gestation.

    E May be congenital.

40► **There is an increased risk of ovarian cancer associated with**

    A Nulliparity.

    B Breast cancer.

    C Prolonged oral contraceptive use.

    D Social class V.

    E Hormone replacement therapy use.

41► **Vaginal *Candida* infection**

    A Is the commonest of all infection during pregnancy.

    B Can be reduced by washing underwear at temperatures greater than 80°C.

    C Is more common during the proliferative phase of the menstrual cycle.

    D Inadequate therapy is the most likely cause of chronic infections.

    E Is more common in women using the progesterone-only pill.

42► Endometriosis
A Is a recognized cause of recurrent miscarriage.
B Is rare after the birth of a first child.
C Is always associated with painful menstruation.
D Should respond to treatment with Provera 30 mg a day.
E Is associated with a higher incidence of endometrial cancer in later life.

43► Following a vaginal hysterectomy without a repair, a woman should be advised
A Not to drive for six weeks.
B That any vaginal bleeding will stop after two weeks.
C That she will need to stay in hospital for at least five days.
D That she will have a vaginal pack and urinary catheter for three days following the operation.
E That she will need a vaginal vault smear after one year.

44► Transvaginal ultrasound of the pelvis
A Requires a full bladder.
B Should not be performed in a woman who is menstruating.
C Can detect a foetal heart at six weeks' gestation.
D Should not be performed in a woman with suspected genital herpes.
E Can accurately diagnose deposits of endometriosis.

45► When prescribing the combined oral contraceptive pill
A Mothers who are not breast feeding should be advised to wait at least six weeks after delivery before starting the pill.
B One should advise that if a pill is missed, provided it is not more than 24 hours late, it can be taken and the packet continued without the risk of pregnancy.
C Barrier contraception is needed for the first 14 days when starting the first pill packet.
D It can be started on the first day after a first trimester termination.
E A previous history of cervical intraepithelial neoplasia is a contraindication.

46► Recurrent miscarriage
A The risk of miscarriage rises after the age of 35 years.
B Over half the cases are associated with anovulatory cycles.
C Progesterone support is of proven benefit.
D Congenital uterine abnormalities account for 15% of cases.
E Parental karyotyping should be performed.

47➤ Dysfunctional uterine bleeding

A In the majority of cases is associated with anovulatory cycles.

B Is improved by a therapeutic dilation of the cervix and curettage of the uterine cavity.

C May be helped by ethamsylate.

D May be associated with leiomyoma.

E Should be considered a relative contraindication to fitting a standard intrauterine contraceptive device.

48➤ In vitro fertilization (IVF)

A Is associated with a multiple pregnancy rate of 14–24%.

B The success rate is the same for a 32-year-old as it is for a 40-year-old.

C Egg collection requires laparoscopy.

D Is associated with a lower incidence of congenital abnormalities than spontaneous pregnancies.

E Legally, no more than three embryos can be transferred at any one time.

49➤ Conservative management strategies for genuine stress incontinence include

A Plevnick vaginal cones.

B Frewen's bladder drill.

C Interferential therapy.

D Hydrotherapy.

E Pelvic floor exercises.

50➤ A tubal pregnancy may be associated with

A Previous ectopic pregnancy.

B Ovulation early in the cycle.

C In vitro fertilization and embryo transfer.

D Previous sterilization.

E Depo-Provera.

51➤ The following syndromes or lesions are correctly paired with a recognized clinical association

A Choriocarcinoma – hyperthyroidism.

B Anorexia nervosa – low basal LH concentration.

C Acute retention of urine – haemorrhoidectomy.

D Hypertension – the administration of bromocriptine.

E The testicular feminization syndrome – hirsutism.

QUESTIONS

52➤ An enterocoele
A Is a true hernia.
B Can be congenital.
C Is caused by an inverted vagina.
D Is associated with dyskexia.
E Is a recognized complication of vaginal hysterectomy.

53➤ Cervical intraepithelial neoplasia (CIN) 3 is characterized by
A Invasion through the basement membrane.
B Spontaneous remission during pregnancy.
C A smear containing dyskaryotic cells.
D A bloodstained vaginal discharge.
E Full thickness loss of stratification and polarity in the epithelium.

54➤ Injectable progestogens used for contraceptive purposes
A Include medroxyprogesterone acetate.
B Can cause irregular vaginal bleeding.
C May cause amenorrhoea.
D Carry a risk of venous thrombosis.
E Are contraindicated in women with hypertension.

55➤ A negative progestogen challenge test
A Suggests low endogenous oestrogen levels.
B Indicates that clomiphene is a suitable drug to induce ovulation.
C Would be expected in cases of primary ovarian failure.
D Would be expected in amenorrhoea associated with anorexia nervosa.
E Is typical of hyperprolactinaemic amenorrhoea.

56➤ Acute retention of urine in the female has a recognized association with
A Haemorrhoidectomy.
B The cauda equina syndrome.
C Incarceration of uterine fibroid.
D Upper motor neurone lesions of the central nervous system.
E Third-degree uterovaginal prolapse.

57➤ Pelvic endometriosis is characteristically associated with
A Vaginal adenosis.
B Hydronephrosis.
C Rectal bleeding.
D Prolonged use of an intrauterine contraceptive device.
E Haematometra.

58► Recognized causes of postmenopausal bleeding include
A Preinvasive carcinoma of the cervix.
B Benign teratoma of the ovary.
C Atrophic vaginitis.
D Subserous fibroids.
E Hepatic cirrhosis.

59► Uterine curettage
A Is associated with an increased incidence of placenta praevia in subsequent pregnancies.
B Has a recognized association with implantation endometriosis.
C By suction curette, is likely to produce histological artifacts.
D Is essential in the investigation of secondary amenorrhoea.
E Is curative in about 50% of cases of menorrhagia of unknown aetiology.

60► Hysteroscopy
A Cannot be performed during a period.
B Requires administration of a general anaesthetic.
C Can be used to locate an endometrial polyp.
D Should not be performed in a woman with a past history of pelvic inflammatory disease.
E Is mandatory in the investigation of a 35-year-old woman presenting with intermenstrual bleeding.

1► **True:** A, B, C
False: D, E

Voluntary effort is not essential; a paraplegic woman can have a normal delivery.

2► **True:** A, B, C, E
False: D

Most candidates answered false to part C, but the presence of a placenta praevia increases the incidence of malpresentation including a face presentation.

3► **True:** A, D, E
False: B, C

Watch for the missed zero in question B which makes it false. It is essential to read the question carefully; 18% of candidates fell into the trap. Symptomatic infections occur in 1–2% of pregnancies and are more common in primigravidae.

4► **True:** A
False: B, C, D, E

A maternal, not paternal, first-degree relative is a high-risk feature. Again, foetal macrosomia, not foetal microsomia, and polyhydramnios are high-risk features for abnormal glucose tolerance.

5► **True:** C, E
False: A, B, D

Every pregnant woman is screened for syphilis, therefore this is a fair question. Wassermann reaction and VDRL are not specific tests and with successful treatment they usually become negative. The reason for continued screening is that early treatment can protect the foetus.

6► **True:** A, B, D, E
False: C

Syphilis, rubella, cytomegalovirus, toxoplasmosis, human immunodeficiency virus and parvovirus are the most important infections that cross the placenta.

ANSWERS AND COMMENTS

7► **True:** C, D
False: A, B, E

Binovular twins are more common in tall women, a piece of useless information.

8► **True:** D
False: A, B, C, E

Defined as a death occurring within 42 days. Again, watch for the missing zero in part B.

9► **True:** B, C
False: A, D, E

Pregnancy-induced hypertension/pre-eclampsia is the commonest cause of maternal death. Parts B, D and E were answered incorrectly by 35% of candidates.

10► **True:** A, C
False: B, D, E

Surprisingly, just under 50% answered part A as false.

11► **True:** C, E
False: A, B, D

Erb's palsy follows damage to C5 and C6 and is usually caused by hyperextension of the neck laterally during shoulder dystocia. Damage to C7 and C8 (Klumpke's palsy) is caused by hyperextension of the arm during a breech delivery. This question was poorly answered.

12► **True:** B, C, D
False: A, E

Congenital dislocation of the hips is four times more common among girls. Most will be successfully treated by splints in 6–12 weeks. Less than 10% will require surgical correction.

13► **True:** B, D
False: A, C, E

Women require an additional 500 kcal a day. Normally 10% of dietary iron is absorbed but this increases to 20% during pregnancy. Iron can only be absorbed in the ferrous state.

14► **True:** A, B, D
False: C, E

The β subunit is immunologically specific. About 15% of candidates fell into the trap. Read the question!

15► **True:** A, B, C, D, E

Apart from part C, this question was very well answered.

16► **True:** A, B, E
False: C, D

The incidence of placental abruption increases with parity. There is an unexplained association between a raised α-fetoprotein (AFP) at 16 weeks and later placental abruption. While a threatened miscarriage can cause a raised AFP, it does not increase the risk of placental abruption later.

17► **True:** A, E
False: B, C, D

The presence of pre-eclampsia may lead to early delivery to avoid complications; it is not spontaneous and this is the key word in the stem. Gestational diabetes is associated with polyhydramnios which may lead to preterm delivery but diabetes itself does not cause preterm labour. This is an example of reading too much into the question.

18► **True:** A, B, E
False: C, D

C and D are included to pad out the question. They are clearly false.

19► **True:** B, C, D
False: A, E

Umbilical cord prolapse complicates one in 300 deliveries. The incidence is increased with any malpresentation. Spasm from cooling is the main cause of foetal distress. Never say never for part E!

20► **True:** A, B, E
False: C, D

Glomerular filtration rate increases by 40%. The vital capacity decreases due to splinting of the diaphragm.

ANSWERS AND COMMENTS

21➤ True: A, B, C
False: D, E

Drug groups lend themselves to this type of question. There are no real tips. One has to draw on one's knowledge.

22➤ True: B, D, E
False: A, C

Babies at 32 weeks do not have the ability to produce meconium.

23➤ True: B, D
False: A, C, E

A, C and E all classically lead to polyhydramnios.

24➤ True: A, B, D, E
False: C

Transplacental haemorrhage may occur, therefore all rhesus-negative mothers should receive anti-D.

25➤ True: B, D
False: A, C, E

Ulcerative colitis classically leads to diarrhoea, not vomiting.

26➤ True: B, E
False: A, C, D

Neural tube defects are diagnosed by ultrasound. There is a significant risk of placental mosaicism with CVS. This is one of the main disadvantages as one fails to get a definitive diagnosis.

27➤ True: B, D
False: A, C, E

Bicornuate uterus is associated with preterm labour but not because the cervix is incompetent.

ANSWERS AND COMMENTS

28► **True:** A, B, E
False: C, D

Babies born to diabetic mothers are more at risk of polycythaemia and hypoglycaemia.

29► **True:** A, C, D
False: B, E

60% of breech babies will be frank or extended at 38 weeks. The incidence of footling breech increases with increased parity.

30► **True:** C, E
False: A, B, D

This type of information is commonly used for MCQs.

31► **True:** A, C, D
False: B, E

Expulsion most commonly occurs with the first period. Only 30% answered this correctly. If the strings cannot be identified, a pelvic ultrasound should be performed to see if the coil is still in the uterus. A woman who has expelled a coil may well not want another fitted, but this is not a contraindication.

32► **True:** A, B, D, E
False: C

It is important to take a male drug history in cases of infertility, especially in those with poor sperm counts.

33► **True:** A, C, D, E
False: B

It is the low vaginal pH that protects against infection. All the others are part of the natural defence mechanisms.

34► **True:** A, B, D, E
False: C

High-dose broad-spectrum antibiotics should be given before an evacuation is performed.

ANSWERS AND COMMENTS

35▶ True: **A, E**
False: **B, C, D**

Pregnancies have been reported following endometrial ablation. The procedure may be performed as a day case, though it is not usual.

36▶ True: **B, C, D, E**
False: **A**

Hyperemesis may occur as early as seven weeks.

37▶ True: **B, C, D**
False: **A, E**

Pethidine is a short-acting analgesic and therefore would not be used for pain control in women with terminal cancer. Lymphoedema is a feature of vulval cancer, not cervical cancer.

38▶ True: **A, C, E**
False: **B, D**

The incidence increases after the menopause.

39▶ True: **E**
False: **A, B, C, D**

Cervical incompetence is associated with second-trimester miscarriages. It can be diagnosed by hysterosalpingogram. Large loop excision of the transformation zone does not appear to predispose to cervical incompetence. Circlage is performed after 12 weeks when first-trimester miscarriages have already occurred.

40▶ True: **A, B**
False: **C, D, E**

Prolonged use of the oral contraceptive pill protects against ovarian carcinoma. It is more common among social classes I and II. Hormone replacement therapy does not appear to increase the risk.

41▶ True: **A, B, D**
False: **C, E**

Almost 40% of pregnant women will demonstrate asymptomatic vaginal colonization. The growth of *Candida* is increased at the end of the luteal phase. Oestrogen-containing oral contraceptives predispose to *Candida* infection.

ANSWERS AND COMMENTS

42➤ True: D
False: A, B, C, E

While endometriosis may improve following a pregnancy, it commonly recurs. Many cases are asymptomatic and are diagnosed during a laparoscopy performed for another indication.

43➤ False: A, B, C, D, E

Vaginal hysterectomy is increasingly being regarded as a minimally invasive procedure. Patients may be discharged after 24–48 hours.

44➤ True: C
False: A, B, D, E

One of the advantages of transvaginal ultrasound is that it does not require a full bladder. It can be performed during menstruation or during vaginal bleeding from a miscarriage. The transvaginal ultrasound can detect a foetal heart from 5 weeks' gestation onwards.

45➤ True: D
False: A, B, C, E

A significant number of women who do not breast feed will ovulate before their six-week postnatal visit. They should be advised to start the combined oral contraceptive pill 14–21 days following delivery. Barrier contraception is required for seven days if the pill is started on the first day of a period.

46➤ True: A, B, E
False: C, D

B caused confusion. Candidates assumed that all cycles were anovulatory and hence a woman could not become pregnant. In fact, she will ovulate occasionally. Congenital uterine abnormality accounts for 5%. Karyotyping should be performed to look for balanced translocations.

47➤ True: C, E
False: A, B, D

Dysfunctional bleeding by definition is diagnosed when no cause can be found. Hence, anovulation and leiomyoma are false. A curettage is a diagnostic procedure. An intrauterine contraception device is associated with an increased menstrual blood loss. A Mirena IUD could be used here. One would not normally fit a standard IUD in a woman who already has heavy periods.

ANSWERS AND COMMENTS

48▶ True: A, E
False: B, C, D

The success falls significantly after the age of 38 years. Egg collection can be performed using vaginal ultrasound-guided needle aspiration. Local anaesthesia and sedation are used.

49▶ True: A, C, E
False: B, D

Frewen's bladder drill is treatment of detrusor instability. Hydrotherapy is a red herring!

50▶ True: A, C, D
False: B, E

A woman who has had a tubal pregnancy has about a 5–7% risk of recurrence in a subsequent pregnancy. Five percent of pregnancies resulting from in vitro fertilization are tubal. About 30% of pregnancies associated with failed sterilization occur in the tube.

51▶ True: A, B, C
False: D, E

This type of association question is sometimes used in college MCQs. Bromocriptine is associated with hypotension.

52▶ True: A, B, E
False: C, D

An enterocoele is caused by herniation of the pouch of Douglas, not vaginal inversion.

53▶ True: C, E
False: A, B, D

Invasion through the basement membrane signifies invasive carcinoma. CIN 3 is asymptomatic and does not present with bloodstained discharge.

54▶ True: A, B, C
False: D, E

Both irregular bleeding and amenorrhoea can occur following an injection of Depo-Provera (medroxyprogesterone acetate 150 mg, aqueous suspension). Venous thrombosis and hypertension are associated with the combined pill and not Depo-Provera.

ANSWERS AND COMMENTS

55► **True:** **A, C, D, E**
False: **B**

Progesterone needs an oestrogenized endometrium to act upon.

56► **True:** **A, C, E**
False: **B, D**

B and D cause urinary incontinence.

57► **False:** **A, B, C, D, E**

Pelvic endometriosis can rarely be associated with hydronephrosis and rectal bleeding but these are not characteristically associated with it.

58► **True:** **C**
False: **A, B, D, E**

Hepatic cirrhosis may lead to clotting disorders which could possibly lead to postmenopausal bleeding but really this is pushing it too far!

59► **True:** **A, B**
False: **C, D, E**

This is a difficult question but curettage is a very common procedure.

60► **True:** **C**
False: **A, B, D, E**

If a woman is bleeding, a hysteroscopy using saline rather than gas as the distension medium may be undertaken. An outpatient hysteroscopy using a paracervical block can be performed. A 35-year-old presenting with intermenstrual bleeding is more likely to have a hormonal cause than endometrial pathology. It would be reasonable to try the combined pill for three months to see if the bleeding settled.

QUESTIONS

1► Asymptomatic bacteriuria

A Occurs in about 5% of women.
B Has a higher incidence among primigravidae.
C Is associated with acute pyelonephritis in 30% of cases.
D Is associated with structural abnormalities of the urinary tract in 15% of cases.
E The most common organism grown is *Escherichia coli*.

2► Rubella infection

A Rapidly crosses the placenta.
B May lead to cataracts in the foetus.
C May cause thrombocytopenia in the foetus.
D Can be confirmed by a foetal blood sample to detect IgG antibodies.
E Can be confirmed by chorionic villus sampling at ten weeks' gestation.

3► Human immunodeficiency virus (HIV)

A Is a retrovirus.
B Asymptomatic infection has no significant effect on pregnancy complication.
C Does not influence the mode of delivery.
D About 15% of babies will remain HIV positive at six months of age.
E Can be isolated from cervical secretions.

4► Postnatal blues

A Usually start between day 3 and day 5.
B May be prolonged by anaemia.
C Are more common among women who have a normal delivery.
D Are prevented by night sedation.
E Occur most often in women discharged early from hospital.

5► Established diabetics who become pregnant are at increased risk of

A Having a baby with congenital abnormalities.
B Developing pregnancy-induced hypertension.
C Delivery by caesarean section.
D Developing oligohydramnios.
E Rapidly progressive retinopathy.

6► Signs of respiratory distress in the newborn include
A Tachypnoea > 60 breaths / min.
B Expiratory grunting.
C Subcostal recession.
D Cyanosis.
E Nasal flaring.

7► The following are autosomal dominant conditions
A Tay–Sachs disease.
B Huntington's chorea.
C Marfan syndrome.
D Phenylketonuria.
E Polyposis coli.

8► High serum α-fetoprotein may be associated with the presence of foetal
A Glucose-6-phosphate dehydrogenase deficiency.
B Down syndrome.
C Turner syndrome.
D Cystic fibrosis.
E Posterior urethral valves.

9► The following drugs are contraindicated during pregnancy
A Captopril.
B Metronidazole.
C Clindamycin vaginal cream.
D Tetracycline.
E Thyroxine.

10► The following should be considered absolute contraindications to attempting external cephalic version
A Rhesus-negative mother.
B Polyhydramnios.
C Pregnancy-induced hypertension.
D Asthmatic mother.
E Diabetic mother.

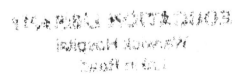

11➤ Factors associated with an increased risk of pulmonary embolism include

A Sickle cell disease.

B Blood group O.

C Obesity.

D Amniocentesis.

E Primigravida.

12➤ Recognized complications of epidural analgesia during labour include

A Dural tap.

B Hypertension.

C Urinary retention.

D Foetal tachycardia.

E Forceps delivery.

13➤ The following provide an accurate assessment of placental function antenatally

A Urinary oestradiol.

B Liquor volume assessment.

C Human placental lactogen.

D Foetal movement charts.

E Umbilical artery Doppler blood flow studies.

14➤ Rhesus isoimmunization

A All rhesus-negative people have 'd' in each half of the genotype.

B Anti-D immunoglobulin 500 IU can eliminate up to 8 ml of Rh-D positive blood from the maternal circulation.

C Maternal IgG crosses the placenta and will cause a foetal haemolytic anaemia.

D Tends to become less severe in successive pregnancies.

E Most commonly follows failure to give prophylaxis.

15➤ Recognized causes of a high head at term include

A Negro mothers.

B Deflexed head.

C Uterine fibroid.

D Previous caesarean section.

E Polyhydramnios.

371

16► A third-degree tear at delivery

A Extends to involve the anal mucosa.

B May follow shoulder dystocia.

C Should be repaired using local infiltration of 0.5% lignocaine.

D The perineal body should be repaired first.

E Following repair, the mother should be placed on a high-residue diet.

17► Cytomegalovirus (CMV)

A Is the commonest primary viral infection of pregnancy in the UK.

B Presentation is usually subclinical.

C Is similar to rubella, only the primary infection causes foetal problems.

D Infection may lead to foetal optic atrophy.

E The virus is not expressed in breast milk.

18► The following are recognized complications of a vacuum delivery

A Cephalohaematoma.

B Facial nerve palsy.

C Vaginal trauma.

D Detachment of the vacuum cup.

E Fracture of foetal skull bones.

19► Iron-deficiency anaemia

A May give rise to a normochromic anaemia.

B May be associated with a reticulocytosis.

C Is more common in multiple pregnancies.

D Increases the risk of postpartum haemorrhage.

E If severe, may be a contraindication to providing an epidural during labour.

20► Neonatal jaundice

A Is associated with raised levels of conjugated bilirubin.

B Occurs in 50% of well babies in the second or third day of life.

C A bilirubin of 350 µmol/l in a term baby of 3.5 kg weight would require phototherapy.

D Occurs more commonly following a vacuum delivery.

E A raised bilirubin level at nine days would most commonly be associated with infection.

21➤ Complications of placental abruption include

A Postpartum haemorrhage.

B Persistent malpresentation of the foetus.

C Disseminated intravascular coagulation.

D Rapid labour.

E Retained placenta.

22➤ Perinatal mortality rate

A Prematurity is the commonest cause of perinatal mortality.

B Is increased in mothers with sickle cell trait.

C Trebles for the fifth child.

D Is lowest for a primigravida aged between 17 and 21 years.

E In 1990 was 8.2/10 000 total births in England and Wales.

23➤ The placenta and umbilical cord

A At term the umbilical cord is about 50 cm long.

B There are no nerves in the umbilical cord or placenta.

C With a placenta increta the villi penetrate through the myometrium to the peritoneum, making it impossible to separate.

D The placenta consists of 30 lobules packed together.

E The most common cord insertion is the Battledore type.

24➤ The following drugs and adverse effects in pregnancy are paired correctly

A Iodides – foetal hypothyroidism.

B Danazol – virilization of female foetus.

C Glibenclamide – neonatal hyperglycaemia.

D Methyldopa – neonatal hypotension.

E Tetracycline – affects foetal teeth.

25➤ Congenital uterine abnormalities in pregnancy are associated with an increased risk of

A Manual removal of placenta.

B Preterm labour.

C Breech presentation.

D Pre-eclampsia.

E Placenta accreta.

QUESTIONS

26► **A well-controlled epileptic woman taking phenytoin and phenobarbitone presents for contraceptive and preconceptual advice. She should be advised that with her current medication**

    A Contraception using the progesterone-only pill will be as effective as in a non-epileptic woman.

    B There is a risk that the frequency of her fits may increase as pregnancy progresses.

    C There is no increased risk of her baby being born mentally defective.

    D There is an increased chance of cleft palate in the child.

    E There is no increased chance of perinatal loss.

27► **Congenital abnormalities in diabetic pregnancies**

    A Account for about half of the perinatal deaths.

    B Are defects of the central nervous system in the majority of cases.

    C Are more common in women with high HBA1 before conception.

    D Have fallen dramatically in incidence in recent years.

    E Are commoner in non-insulin-dependent diabetes than in insulin-dependent patients.

28► **Prophylactic use of oral iron therapy during pregnancy**

    A Iron absorption during the first trimester is increased compared with the non-pregnant state.

    B Non-compliance occurs in less than 10% of pregnant patients.

    C Gastric side effects are dose related.

    D Is associated with an increase in the maternal MCV.

    E Reduces the incidence of iron-deficiency anaemia in the newborn infant.

29► **When counselling a mother about a home delivery at her booking visit, the following should be regarded as contraindications**

    A Previous breech delivery.

    B Rhesus-negative mother.

    C Shoe size less than three.

    D Well-controlled hyperglycaemia.

    E Previous ectopic pregnancy.

30► **Polyhydramnios**

    A The average volume of liquor at 36 weeks is 1000 ml.

    B Should be considered if foetal parts are difficult to palpate at 34 weeks' gestation.

    C Is associated with foetal bowel atresia.

    D Increases the risk of postpartum haemorrhage.

    E May be treated by paracentesis.

31► Uterine fibroids may be associated with

A Intermenstrual bleeding.

B Genuine stress incontinence.

C Polycythaemia.

D Urinary frequency.

E Delayed involution postpartum.

32► Endometrial carcinoma

A Occurs rarely before the age of 40.

B Is more common among multiparous women.

C Is associated with diabetes.

D Is nearly always squamous in nature.

E Should be treated with radiotherapy in the first instance.

33► Premenstrual tension

A Occurs most frequently around the age of 35 years.

B Sufferers must have a symptom-free window to allow the diagnosis to be made.

C Is associated with high luteal progesterone levels.

D May respond to pyridoxine.

E Should be treated with prothiadine.

34► Predisposing factors to candidal vaginitis include

A Diabetes mellitus.

B Broad-spectrum antibiotics.

C Progesterone-only pill.

D Corticosteroids.

E Intrauterine contraceptive device.

35► Adenomyosis

A May lead to secondary dysmenorrhoea.

B Causes polymenorrhagia.

C Can be diagnosed by endometrial biopsy.

D Causes uterine enlargement.

E May lead to infertility.

36► Polycystic ovarian syndrome classically leads to

A Hirsutism.

B Infertility.

C Premature menopause.

D Dysmenorrhoea.

E Obesity.

QUESTIONS

37► Invasive carcinoma of the vulva

A The mean age of affected women is 80 years.

B Is more common in multiparous women.

C Is squamous in 90% of cases.

D Is preceded by cervical intraepithelial neoplasia in up to 30% of cases.

E Most commonly occurs in the labia minora.

38► The following are absolute contraindications to use of the combined oral contraceptive pill

A Diabetes.

B Oligomenorrhoea.

C Previous thromboembolism.

D Carcinoma of the colon.

E Women over the age of 40.

39► Increased risk of ectopic (tubal) pregnancy is associated with

A Vasectomy.

B Tubal ligature.

C Danazol.

D Clomiphene citrate.

E Reversal of sterilization.

40► Detrusor instability

A Is the commonest cause of urinary incontinence.

B May occur following a colposuspension for the first time.

C Pelvic floor exercises are the first line of management.

D May improve with the use of ditropan.

E Can be diagnosed accurately using a free flow rate.

41► Ovulation may be confirmed by

A Basal body temperature recording.

B Positive postcoital test.

C Proliferative phase endometrial biopsy.

D Pelvic ultrasound performed on day 10 of the cycle.

E Luteal phase plasma oestradiol.

QUESTIONS

42➤ The following doses of progesterone provide endometrial protection if given for 12 days each cycle with continuous oestrogen to a postmenopausal woman

A 10 mg medroxyprogesterone.

B 150 µg norgestrol.

C 1 mg norethisterone.

D 350 µg norethisterone.

E 30 µg levonorgestrel.

43➤ Danazol

A Reduces high-density lipoproteins.

B Increases oestradiol levels.

C Suppresses ovulation.

D May cause acne.

E May be associated with voice changes.

44➤ The following are risk factors for developing osteoporosis

A Early menopause.

B Negro race.

C Steroid therapy.

D Obesity.

E Cigarette smoking.

45➤ The following may give rise to postmenopausal bleeding

A Cervical intraepithelial neoplasia.

B Endometrial polyp.

C Vulval dystrophy.

D Treatment with tibolone.

E Continuous combined hormone replacement therapy.

46➤ Recommended treatments for amenorrhoea include

A Danazol.

B Progesterone-only pill.

C Clomiphene citrate.

D Cyclokapron.

E Mefenamic acid.

47➤ A cervical ectropion

A Is more common among women taking the oral contraceptive pill.
B Is a true ulcer.
C May lead to a postcoital bleeding.
D Is frequently associated with cervical intraepithelial neoplasia.
E Is common in postmenopausal women.

48➤ Dyspareunia may commonly be caused by

A Pelvic inflammatory disease.
B Mittelschmerz.
C Irritable bowel syndrome.
D Cervical polyps.
E Retroverted uterus.

49➤ Hydatidiform mole

A Occurs more commonly in the Far East.
B Most complete moles have 46 XX karyotype.
C May present with early pre-eclampsia.
D Some 1% go on to develop trophoblastic malignancy.
E A woman with a benign mole has a 10% chance of a repeat mole in another pregnancy and so should have an early ultrasound scan in the next pregnancy.

50➤ Relative contraindications to HRT include

A Moderate hypertension.
B Heavy cigarette smoking.
C Hyperlipidaemia.
D Varicose veins.
E Otosclerosis.

51➤ Cone biopsy of the cervix

A Is associated with an increased incidence of infertility.
B Is most commonly performed using a laser.
C Should be performed just before the start of a menstrual period.
D May lead to cervical stenosis and dysmenorrhoea.
E Should not be performed if invasive carcinoma is suspected because of the increased risk of tumour spread.

52➤ Carcinoma of the uterine cervix

A Is typically squamous in nature.

B Characteristically originates at the squamocolumnar junction.

C Is more common in nulliparous women.

D Typically metastasizes to the superficial inguinal lymph nodes.

E May lead to ureteric obstruction.

53➤ Recognized causes of vaginal discharge in a ten-year-old who has not started her periods include

A Systemic corticosteroid therapy.

B A foreign body in the vagina.

C Threadworms.

D Dysgerminoma of the ovary.

E Ectopic ureter.

54➤ Norplant

A Consists of five rods each inserted into the inner aspect of the upper arm.

B Is more effective in obese women.

C Should be removed after five years.

D There is frequently a delay in return of fertility following removal similar to that seen with Depo-Provera.

E Plasma progesterone levels are similar to those achieved with the progesterone-only pill.

55➤ Progesterone-containing IUCD (Mirena)

A Is less effective than the Novogard IUCD.

B Leads to amenorrhoea in 60% of women within six months of insertion.

C Requires a paracervical block for insertion.

D Is effective for seven years.

E Is associated with an increased risk of tubal pregnancy compared to a Nova-T.

56➤ Infertility caused by tubal damage

A Accounts for 10% of cases of primary infertility.

B Is most commonly caused by chlamydial infection.

C May follow a suction termination of pregnancy.

D May be diagnosed by an air insufflation test.

E May be treated by ovulation induction and intrauterine insemination.

57► Surgery for stress incontinence of urine

A Aims to elevate the bladder neck above the pelvic diaphragm.

B Should only be performed if the diagnosis has been confirmed by urodynamic assessment.

C May lead to voiding difficulties.

D Can be associated with detrusor instability postoperatively.

E Has a success rate of 85% associated with an anterior vaginal colporrhaphy.

58► Following a laparoscopic sterilization

A A woman should not return to work for ten days.

B Contraception should be continued until the next menstrual period in all cases.

C A woman should be warned that her menstrual periods will be heavier.

D There is a failure rate of greater than one in 1000 cases.

E A third of those women who conceive will have a tubal pregnancy.

59► Radiotherapy for cervical carcinoma

A Leads to vaginal stenosis in 80% of women.

B Is associated with a 40% five-year survival for stage II disease.

C Can lead to vesicovaginal fistulae.

D Leads to a premature menopause for which hormone replacement therapy is contraindicated.

E Should not be given following a Wertheim hysterectomy.

60► A retroverted uterus

A Occurs in over 25% of women.

B Is associated with an increased incidence of infertility.

C Is associated with acute retention of urine in pregnancy.

D Can be corrected using a Hodge pessary.

E If fixed, is an indication to perform a ventrosuspension.

ANSWERS AND COMMENTS

1▶ True: A, C, E
False: B, D

Asymptomatic bacteriuria increases with parity and age. It is associated with structural abnormalities of the renal tract in only 3–5% of cases.

2▶ True: A, B, C, E
False: D

Rubella infection may lead to hepatosplenomegaly with thrombocytopenia if the mother is infected in the last half of pregnancy. Infection may be confirmed by foetal blood sample but it is IgM antibodies that are looked for. Electron microscopy and modern immune methods may be able to determine if the virus has crossed the placenta on a chorionic villus sample performed between eight and 11 weeks. Part E was correctly answered by 20% of candidates.

3▶ True: A, B, D, E
False: C

There is a little evidence that asymptomatic HIV infection has any significant effect on the pregnancy complications; 40% of candidates answered B correctly. HIV can be isolated from cervical secretions.

4▶ True: A, B, D
False: C, E

Postnatal blues are more common among women who stay in hospital. Forceps deliveries tend to stay longer, hence are more likely to suffer from the blues. A good night's sleep helps to reduce the incidence and hence the benefit of night sedation.

5▶ True: A, B, C, E
False: D

Retinopathy does not usually progress rapidly but occasionally can do so. Most candidates scored 5 for this section.

6▶ True: A, B, C, D, E

This question was well answered.

7▶ True: B, C
False: A, D, E

This type of information is commonly used for MCQ papers. It is worth looking up a list the day before the exam.

8▶ True: C, E
False: A, B, D

Down syndrome is associated with a low α-fetoprotein.

9▶ True: A, D
False: B, C, E

Metronidazole and clindamycin cream have both been used to treat bacterial vaginosis during pregnancy. Tetracycline is associated with staining of the teeth.

10▶ False: A, B, C, D, E

A rhesus-negative mother should be given anti-D immunoglobulin following external cephalic version. Version may well not be successful in cases of polyhydramnios but it can be attempted. Note the stem is a *double* negative, i.e. none of the listed is an absolute contraindication.

11▶ True: A, C
False: B, D, E

Factors associated with an increased risk are increasing age and parity, obesity, confinement to bed, delivery by caesarean section, blood group other than O, sickle cell disease.

12▶ True: A, C, E
False: B, D

Epidurals are associated with hypotension.

13▶ True: B, E
False: A, C, D

There is no totally accurate method of assessing the placental function during the antenatal period. Measurement of liquor volume and umbilical artery Doppler blood studies are the most accurate available. Serial urinary oestradiol estimations, though cumbersome, may be of value. Single readings are not. Foetal movement charts do not give an accurate assessment of foetal wellbeing.

ANSWERS AND COMMENTS

14▶ True: A, C, E
False: B, D

500 IU immunoglobulin can eliminate 4 ml/g Rh-D positive blood. Rhesus isoimmunoglobulin tends to become more severe in successive pregnancies.

15▶ True: A, B, C, E
False: D

Most candidates answered true to D but while a caesarean section may be necessary if the head fails to descend into the pelvis during labour, it does not cause the head to remain high.

16▶ True: A, B
False: C, D, E

One should provide better analgesia than local for repair of a third-degree tear. The anal mucosa should be repaired first, followed by repair of the sphincter, then the perineal body. The mother should be placed on a low-residue diet.

17▶ True: A, B, D
False: C, E

Congenital infection follows primary infection in 75% of cases and reinfection in 25%. About 75% of women who acquire CMV in pregnancy will be immune at the time. About 5% have a seriously damaged infant.

18▶ True: A, C, D
False: B, E

Facial nerve palsy and fractured skull are complications of a forceps delivery.

19▶ True: A, C
False: B, D, E

The provision of iron in cases of anaemia may be associated with a reticulocytosis. A low platelet count is a contraindication to an epidural. Anaemia does not increase the risk of postpartum haemorrhage occurring, but may increase the risk associated with haemorrhage if it occurs.

20➤ True: B, C, D, E
False: A

Neonatal jaundice is associated with raised levels of unconjugated bilirubin. The level to treat varies with different hospitals but a bilirubin level of about 300 μmol/l in a well baby of 3.5 kg weight is usually treated with phototherapy. It is more common following a vacuum delivery because of the reabsorption of the cephalohaematoma.

21➤ True: A, C, D
False: B, E

Placental abruption tends to make the uterus more irritable and hence labour more rapid. The associated blood loss can lead to disseminated intravascular coagulation and hence postpartum haemorrhage.

22➤ True: A
False: B, C, D, E

Seventy percent of neonatal deaths are associated with prematurity. The denominator for perinatal mortality is 1000, not 10 000. Read the question carefully – 25% of candidates fell into this trap at the last validation.

23➤ True: A, B, E
False: C, D

With placenta increta the villi penetrate into the myometrium but it is a placenta percreta in which the villi penetrate into the peritoneal covering. The placenta consists of 15–20 lobules packed together.

24➤ True: A, B, E
False: C, D

Glibenclamide taken during pregnancy will lead to neonatal hypoglycaemia. Methyldopa does not have any effect on neonatal blood pressure.

25➤ True: A, B, C
False: D, E

Uterine abnormalities are associated with malpresentation, particularly transverse lie.

ANSWERS AND COMMENTS

26➤ True: A, B, D
False: C, E

A refers to the progesterone-only pill. The question would be false for the combined oral contraceptive pill. Antiepileptics compete and higher doses are needed for the same degree of efficacy (hepatic enzyme recruitment). The incidence of fit may increase as pregnancy progresses. As the plasma volume increases, the plasma concentration of antiepileptics falls. Frequently the dose required increases. Even epileptic women who are not on medication have a higher incidence of congenital abnormalities and perinatal loss.

27➤ True: A, C
False: B, D, E

Congenital abnormalities are increased threefold in insulin-dependent diabetes. Good control, i.e. a low HBA1 before conception, reduces the incidence. Diet or tablet-controlled diabetics are not at particular increased risk of congenital abnormalities.

28➤ True: C, D
False: A, B, E

Because of the side effects associated with iron, the non-compliance rate is much higher than 10%.

29➤ False: A, B, C, D, E

None of these could be considered a contraindication to a safe home delivery. A previous breech delivery has no bearing on this pregnancy; indeed, a previous successful vaginal breech delivery would be a good prognostic indicator. Most candidates felt shoe size less than three was a contraindication, but most women with shoe size less than three deliver vaginally. The woman must be judged as a whole – her general shape and frame and the size of the baby. Shoe size is a very soft indicator of pelvic size.

30➤ True: A, B, C, D, E

Apart from A, the answers are logical. Despite this, candidates answered poorly.

ANSWERS AND COMMENTS

31► **True:** A, C, D, E
    False: B

A pedunculated fibroid within the endometrial cavity can give rise to intermenstrual bleeding. Polycythaemia is a rare but recognized complication of fibroids.

32► **True:** A, C
    False: B, D, E

Only 2% of cases present before the age of 40. Total abdominal hysterectomy and bilateral salpingo-oophorectomy should be used as first-line therapy.

33► **True:** A, B, C, D
    False: E

PMT occurs in ovulatory cycles and therefore is associated with high luteal progesterone. Tranquillizers should be avoided in the main. More recently, Prozac (fluoxetine) has been used successfully.

34► **True:** A, B, D
    False: C, E

The combined pill predisposes but not the progesterone-only pill.

35► **True:** A, D
    False: B, C, E

Adenomyosis may lead to heavy periods but not more frequent (polymenorrhagia) periods. One needs a myometrial biopsy to diagnose adenomyosis.

36► **True:** A, B, E
    False: C, D

The classic presentation of polycystic ovarian syndrome (PCO) is amenorrhoea, infertility, obesity and hirsutism (Stein–Leventhal syndrome). While PCO is associated with amenorrhoea, it does not lead to an early menopause.

37► **True:** C, D
    False: A, B, E

The mean age of affected women is 60 years. The most common site is the labia majora.

38► **True:** C
False: A, B, D, E

Care needs to be exercised when giving the combined pill to a woman over 40, but age alone is not an *absolute* contraindication.

39► **True:** B, E
False: A, C, D

A significant number of the pregnancies occurring following sterilization are tubal.

40► **True:** B, D
False: A, C, E

Genuine stress incontinence is the commonest cause of urinary leakage. There is a 10% incidence of de novo detrusor instability following a colposuspension. Pelvic floor excercises are used to treat stress incontinence primarily. They can be used for instability in conjunction with anti-cholinergics and bladder retraining. Detrusor instability can only be diagnosed accurately with filling cystometry.

41► **True:** A, B
False: C, D, E

A *luteal* phase endometrial biopsy could be used to confirm ovulation. A pelvic ultrasound performed on day 10 may show developing follicles, but one would need to repeat it after suspected ovulation to confirm it had occurred. A luteal phase *progesterone*, not oestradiol, level is required.

42► **True:** A, C
False: B, D, E

This question was poorly answered but this is important information for family doctors to allow them to plan hormone replacement regimens.

43► **True:** A, C, D, E
False: B

Danazol may cause hoarseness in a small number of women, which is permanent. If a woman notices any changes in her voice she should stop the medication at once.

ANSWERS AND COMMENTS

44➤ True: A, C, E
False: B, D

Accepted risk factors include: premature menopause; Caucasian or Asian origin; family history; low body weight; nulliparity; cigarette smoking; high alcohol intake; high caffeine intake; low calcium intake; sedentary lifestyle; prolonged oral steroids; hyperthyroidism.

45➤ True: B, D, E
False: A, C

Continuous combined hormone replacement (i.e. daily oestrogen and progesterone) and Livial are marketed as bleed-free therapy but they both may be associated with postmenopausal bleeding, i.e. irregular bleeding during the settling in phase.

46➤ True: C
False: A, B, D, E

Clomiphene citrate may be used to induce ovulation in a woman with anovulatory amenorrhoea.

47➤ True: A, C
False: B, D, E

A cervical ectropion is a normal finding and should not be overtreated.

48➤ True: A
False: B, C, D, E

The key word is *commonly*. While a large cervical polyp may be associated with dyspareunia, it is not common. Dilated loops of small bowel may cause dyspareunia if prolapsed into the pelvis. Retroverted uteri can cause position-related pain.

49➤ True: A, B, C
False: D, E

Most complete moles are 46 XX karyotype, while incomplete moles are usually triploid 69 XXX or XXY. Up to 10% may develop choriocarcinoma. A woman with a benign mole has a 1–4% chance of a repeat mole in another pregnancy. The second part of the statement is true and is there to put you off.

ANSWERS AND COMMENTS

50➤ True: E
  False: A, B, C, D

There is some evidence that otosclerosis may progress rapidly with oestrogen therapy. Care needs to be exercised in such cases. There is controversy regarding HRT and thrombosis at the time of writing. Currently, varicose veins should not be regarded as a problem.

51➤ True: D
  False: A, B, C, E

Cone biopsy is now most commonly performed using a hot wire loop. It is best performed after a period. It can lead to cervical stenosis in a very small number of cases. Loop cone biopsy is used to obtain tissue for diagnosis in cases of carcinoma of the cervix. It does not increase the risk of spread.

52➤ True: A, B, E
  False: C, D

It is vulval carcinoma that typically metastasizes to the superficial inguinal lymph nodes. Cervical carcinoma spreads to the iliac nodes.

53➤ True: A, B, C, E
  False: D

Foreign body and threadworms are the commonest causes of vaginal discharge in a ten-year-old. Candidates felt that an ectopic ureter would be detected well before the age of ten years but it *is* a recognized cause.

54➤ True: C, E
  False: A, B, D

Norplant consists of six rods. It is less effective in providing contraception for obese women. Fertility returns promptly after removal.

55➤ False: A, B, C, D, E

The Mirena is a more effective contraceptive than the Novogard. It leads to amenorrhoea in up to 40% of women. It has a slightly wider diameter than a standard intrauterine contraceptive device but can be inserted without a paracervical block in a significant number of women. The Mirena is effective for five years.

ANSWERS AND COMMENTS

56➤ True: B, C
False: A, D, E

A tubal factor accounts for about 20% of cases of primary infertility in most published series. Women should be screened for chlamydial infection before a termination of pregnancy to reduce the incidence of pelvic infection. Air insufflation is an old test and is unreliable. It has been replaced by a laparoscopy and dye or a hysterosalpingogram.

57➤ True: A, B, C, D
False: E

All those with an interest in female urinary incontinence feel patients should have urodynamic assessment before surgery. Both voiding difficulties and de novo detrusor instability are side effects of both a colposuspension and a needle suspension. An anterior colporrhaphy is associated with only a 50–60% success rate.

58➤ True: D, E
False: A, B, C

Most women should be able to return to work after 5–7 days. Tubal ligation is effective at once; there is no need to continue contraception following the procedure if it is performed immediately postmenstrually. If performed mid-cycle, there is a risk the patient may have already ovulated. Those women who are taking the oral contraceptive pill should be advised to complete the pack to avoid irregular bleeding. Tubal ligation does not affect periods.

59➤ True: C
False: A, B, D, E

The vaginal stenosis rate used to be in the order of 80% postradiotherapy before the additional use of topical oestrogens. Radiotherapy is associated with a 70–75% five-year survival for stage IIa disease. It causes a premature menopause but hormone replacement therapy is not contraindicated. It can be given following a Wertheim hysterectomy.

60➤ True: C, D
False: A, B, E

A retroverted uterus is found in 15–20% of women. It is not associated with infertility. A retroverted uterus may become incarcerated in the pelvis at about 16 weeks, leading to acute retention of urine. A ventrosuspension is now seldom, if ever, performed as results are rarely permanent. Anyway, the stem referred to *fixed* retroversion. This is usually due to pathology.

Index

Index

Index

Index

Index

Index

Index

397

Index

Index

Index

Index

Index

Index